ic Associ

D1354143

For Churchill Livingstone

Publisher: Timothy Horne
Project Editor: Jane Shanks
Copy Editor: Anita Hible
Project Controller: Kay Hunston
Design Direction: Erik Bigland

MCQs in Paediatrics for the DCH Examination

Antonio A T Chuh MRCGP LRCP (Edin) LRCS (Edin) LRCPS (Glas)
DCH (Lond) DCH (Irel) DCCH (Edin) DPDerm (Wales) Dip G-U Med (Lond)

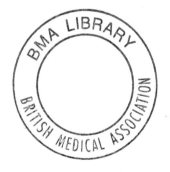

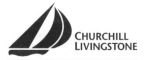

CHURCHILL LIVINGSTONE

EDINBURGH LONDON NEW YORK PHILADELPHIA SAN FRANCISCO SYDNEY TORONTO 1998

CHURCHILL LIVINGSTONE
A Division of Harcourt Brace and Company Limited

Robert Stevenson House, 1–3 Baxter's Place, Leith Walk,
Edinburgh EH1 3AF, UK

First published 1998

ISBN 0 443 06149 1

British Library of Cataloguing in Publication Data
A catalogue record for this book is available from the British
Library.

Library of Congress Cataloging in Publication Data
A catalog record for this book is available from the Library of
Congress.

Medical knowledge is constantly changing. As information
becomes available, changes in treatment, procedures,
equipment and the use of drugs become necessary. The
author and publisher have, as far as it is possible, taken care
to ensure that the information given in the text is accurate
and up-to-date. However, readers are strongly advised to
confirm that the information, especially with regard to drug
usage, complies with current legislation and standard of
practice.

The
publisher's
policy is to use
**paper manufactured
from sustainable forests**

Produced by Addison Wesley Longman China Limited, Hong Kong
EPC/01

CONTENTS

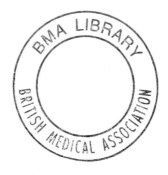

PREFACE

This book is written primarily for candidates taking the Diploma in Child Health examination. It is a collection of 480 multiple choice questions, up to 30% of which are related to community child health issues such as nutrition, growth, development, screening, immunizations, child health promotion, accidents and child abuse. The Royal Colleges are now placing more emphasis upon community and primary care issues, and books covering hospital paediatrics may not treat such topics adequately.

By attempting the questions under strictly timed conditions, the technique to answering MCQ questions can be sharpened. On reading the study notes accompanying the answers, and then referring to standard textbooks, a firm theoretical base for answering questions in other sections of the examination will be established. In addition, the introductory section serves as a personal guide to preparing for the whole examination.

Almost all of the major topics tested in the multiple choice, written, clinical and oral sections of the examinations are covered in some detail in this book. The balance of the individual topics with the level of difficulty is also geared towards the actual examination.

This book will also be useful to candidates preparing for other examinations such as the MRCGP, GP summative assessment, DCCH, DTCH and the MB ChB Finals. Despite revisions, much of the emphasis of the undergraduate syllabus is still on hospital paediatrics. Thus, for medical students, this book will give a more balanced and rounded view on child health care in the community.

I wish to thank all my colleagues, former teachers and examiners who have unwittingly provided ideas for many of the questions. Special thanks are due to Timothy Horne and Jane Shanks of Churchill Livingstone for their support and assistance in the preparation of this book.

A A T Chuh

INTRODUCTION

THE DIPLOMA IN CHILD HEALTH (DCH) EXAMINATIONS

The DCH examinations are intended for medical practitioners entering general practice, community medicine and other types of primary care paediatrics. Knowledge of common diseases of infancy and childhood is tested, but the greatest emphasis is put on community paediatric issues, such as nutrition and feeding, growth and development, immunizations, screening, behavioural problems, child health promotion, health education and preventive paediatrics.

Knowledge of basic sciences such as anatomy, physiology, biochemistry, pharmacology, pathology and microbiology, as related to infancy, childhood and adolescence, is also essential.

The Royal Colleges each have their own regulations and examination formats for the DCH examination.

DCH (London)

This is held by the Royal College of Physicians of London, 11 St Andrew's Place, Regent's Park, London NW1 4LE.

It is recommended that candidates should have at least 6 months paediatric experience. It is held twice yearly in March and October.

The written examination is taken first with a multiple choice question (MCQ) paper and an essay paper. The essay paper usually comprises 10 short essay questions with 2 long case commentaries. Candidates who fail the MCQ paper are not allowed to proceed to the clinical examination, and their essay papers are not marked.

The clinical examination consists of a long case followed by 3 to 6 short cases. In addition, there is a short case specifically designed to test developmental examinations, including vision and hearing tests.

DCH (Glasgow)

This is held by the Royal College of Physicians and Surgeons of Glasgow, 234–242 St Vincent Street, Glasgow G2 5RJ.

Candidates should have graduated in medicine 2 or more years previous to the date of the examination. In addition, candidates must have been in residence, for 6 months or more, as a medical officer in a paediatric hospital post which is recognized by the College. Alternatively, they should have attended with clinical instruction at a children's hospital or the paediatric department of a general hospital for a period of 6 months full time or not less than 12 months part time.

DCH (Ireland)

This is held by the Conjoint Board of the Royal College of Physicians and the Royal College of Surgeons in Ireland. Apply to the Irish Conjoint Board, 123 St Stephen's Green, Dublin 2, Eire.

Candidates should have been in possession of a recognized qualification for not less than 10 months and have held the post of resident medical officer in a recognized children's hospital or in the paediatric department of a recognized general hospital for 6 months, or in a non-recognized hospital for 12 months.

DCH (Dublin)

This is held by the Faculty of Medicine, University College Dublin, Earlsfort Terrace, Dublin 2, Eire.

Candidates must have been either a resident medical officer in a recognized children's hospital for 12 months, or a resident medical officer in a recognized paediatric department of a general hospital for 12 months.

For this examination, attendance at an evening course for 6 weeks before the examination is compulsory.

The Diploma in Community Child Health (DCCH) Examination

The Diploma in Community Child Health (DCCH) examination is held by the Royal College of Physicians of Edinburgh, the Royal College of General Practitioners, and the Faculty of Public Health Medicine of the Royal Colleges of Physicians. Apply to the Royal College of Physicians of Edinburgh, 9 Queen Street, Edinburgh EH2 1JQ.

Candidates should provide a testimonial, signed by a Member or Fellow of one of the Colleges or the Faculty, to certify suitability to take the examination.

An objective, structured clinical examination (OSCE) and a slide test are part of the examination. Videos may also be shown in the slide test.

PREPARING FOR THE DCH EXAMINATION

Multiple Choice Question (MCQ) Paper

The MCQ paper usually consists of 60 questions, each with a stem statement with five following items. The candidate has to answer each item as 'true', 'false' or 'don't know'. As with other postgraduate MCQ papers, 1 mark is awarded for a correct answer, 1 mark is deducted for an incorrect answer and no mark is given for a 'don't know' answer.

As the MCQ paper must be passed before proceeding to the clinical examinations, it is best to spend much time preparing for it. Moreover, most of the written section can be covered while doing MCQ test papers (see later).

It is important to read the questions carefully, as every word is likely to be useful and significant. There is usually no hidden trap. Interpret all the questions at their face meanings.

Remember that each item in the question is independent of other items. Try to think of the question as five separate questions with no link between them.

Studies have repeatedly shown that the more questions attempted, the better is the final score. My habit is therefore to answer all the questions. Many candidates will not have the courage to do this. The most effective strategy is that one should aim at answering as many questions as possible.

The trick to perform well in the MCQ paper is to study a lot of MCQ questions. Thus, the eight papers in this book should be attempted in strictly timed examination conditions, without first looking at the answers.

Once a paper is finished, the final mark can be calculated using the formula:

$$\text{Final score} = \frac{\text{Number of correct answers} - \text{Number of wrong answers}}{3}$$

In this way, a total number of 300 items will give a maximum score of 100. As a rule of thumb, a score of 55–60 should be the target. In reality, the minimum score needed to pass may be a little lower.

The study notes can then be studied in conjunction with standard textbooks. I would recommend that, in addition to this book, four other books should be available for revision: a medium-sized textbook on hospital paediatrics, a textbook on community paediatrics, a book on the child health promotion programme and an updated publication on immunizations.

At 3 to 4 weeks before the examination, questions in this book can be revised by tackling questions again in each discipline by following the subject index. The weaker areas can then be identified and further work done before the examination.

Short essays

It is not difficult to prepare for the short essays. When tackling MCQ questions in this book, always ask yourself the following questions:

1. What is the cause (genetic? environmental?) of the condition?
2. How do children with this condition present?
3. What are the complications? What will I expect to see in the best case and in the worst case?
4. How do I confirm the diagnosis?
5. What are the differential diagnoses?
6. When I am facing a child with such a condition, what treatments (form, route, dose, precautions) should I offer as a first-line management?
7. What if the first line of management does not work?
8. When should I refer? To whom?
9. Can the condition be prevented? (Always think in terms of primary, secondary and tertiary prevention.)
10. How do I help the child and the family in the long term?
11. What implications are there for the development and education of the child?
12. How will the primary health care team be involved in the care of the child and the family?

In studying for postgraduate examinations, the efficiency is usually low if you study a textbook page by page from cover to cover. Thus, by studying an MCQ book and referring to the study notes and textbooks, you will find that the materials are easily memorized.

About 7 to 8 minutes should be spent on each question, thus leaving spare time for the more difficult questions.

As the questions are supposed to be short essays, do not write in note form. Do not write in long paragraphs, as some of the points might be missed by the examiner. Write in short paragraphs, with only 1–2 points in each paragraph. All the relevant points will thus be scored.

My habit is to give headings to the paragraphs, e.g. aetiology, presentation, diagnosis, treatment, prevention. Very little time is needed to do this. With clear headings, I can remember clearly what I am going to write in the 3–4 paragraphs under 'presentation'. I shall remember to leave time for 'diagnosis' and 'treatment' and other headings if needed. I can automatically maintain a good balance of materials in the short essay.

The biggest advantage of using short paragraphs with headings is that such will demonstrate to the examiner that the answer is well organized. The examiner will know where to look for, say, the aetiology and will not miss giving any mark that the answer deserves.

Case commentaries

To prepare for the case commentaries, a familiarity with principles of community paediatrics and resources in the community, especially the primary health care team (PHCT), is needed.

Thus, when coming across relevant questions in this book, refer to the corresponding pages of a textbook on community paediatrics.

Introduction

The concept of the PHCT is central in this paper. List all the possible members of a PHCT. Understand all their job responsibilities and how they work as a team.

Questions in this section usually ask for specific aspects on the management. Try to limit yourself to that specific aspect first and expand to cover other issues if such are relevant.

The following framework will help to organize your answers clearly:

When asked about	Think of
Diagnosis	Diagnoses in physical, psychological and social terms.
Problems	Problems to the child, parents, siblings. Medical and psychosocial problems. Drug compliance. Problems in physical and psychosocial development. Problems in school, future career prospects. Growth and nutritional problems. Immunization problems. Financial problems. Behavioural problems, risk of child abuse, risk of SIDS, risk of accidents. (If appropriate, problems to the PHCT and hospital staff, burden on the society.)
Management	Medical, psychological and social aspects of management. Management offered by the GP and the PHCT, particularly the health visitor and social worker, the paediatrician and other hospital staff. The key worker concept. How to ensure compliance. How to cope with sudden deterioration, complications and death. How to ensure normal schooling, involvement of teachers. Planning for career and marriage prospects. How to ensure continuity of care in the long term.
Child abuse	How to confirm the suspicions (delayed presentation, multiple injuries, classical injuries, evidence given by child, clinical photographs, clotting profiles?). Involvements of PHCT, especially the social worker and health visitor, and NSPCC worker. Emergency Protection Order (who should apply, how, for how long, who can appeal?). Case conference (attended by whom, aims, possible outcome?). Child Protection Register, future role of GP and social worker. Criminal prosecution, likely outcomes. Importance of best interests of the child. Future development and schooling of the child and siblings, behavioural problems.

Sexual abuse	When to suspect? (History volunteered by child, behavioural problems, sexual behaviour inappropriate for age, sexually transmitted diseases? Signs of trauma?).
	When and how to examine (best in presence of genitourinary physician and paediatrician), consent of child, confidentiality issues, swabs for chlamydia, gonorrhoea and trichomoniasis, chain of custody, trace evidence, clinical photographs, notes and diagrams.
	Then follow child abuse plan as above.
Neglect and emotional abuse	When to suspect (non-organic failure to thrive, deprivation hands and feet, frozen watchfulness, radar gaze, deprivation dwarfism, risk factors, developmental delay, behavioural problems).
	Follow child abuse plan as above.
Munchausen syndrome by proxy	When to suspect (must have very high index of suspicion, consult senior colleagues, obtain evidence).
	Ddx (rare syndromes, connective tissue diseases, ddx of pyrexia of unknown origin).
	Variety (e.g. trichotillomania by proxy).
	Underlying or other psychiatric disorders of the carer (usually mother).
	Follow child abuse plan as above.
SIDS	Confirm death.
	Warn parents that police will be involved.
	Allow parents to see baby.
	Autopsy to rule out underlying causes.
	Family history of sudden death / SIDS.
	Care for bereavement (stages, signs of pathological mourning).
	Future prevention (no sleeping in prone position, no overlaying, no overheating, breastfeeding if possible, minimize passive smoking).
	Apnoea alarm (not of proven benefit, for psychological comfort only).
Multiple-handicapped child	Follow 'management' plan above.
	Management offered by GP, social worker, health visitor, district nurse, paediatrician, physiotherapist, occupational therapist, speech therapist, orthoptist, ophthalmologist, audiologist, otolaryngologist, psychologist, paediatric psychiatrist, orthopaedic surgeon, dietician, dentist, normal and special school teachers.
	Education Act 1981 (special educational needs, Statement of Special Needs, reviews, appeals).
Prevention	Primary, secondary and tertiary preventions.

Introduction

Screening as a form of secondary prevention.
Wilson and Jungner's criteria for screening programmes.
Sensitivity, specificity, positive and negative predictive values, yield, incremental yield, cost-effectiveness.
Prevention to decrease incidence and prevalence.
Prevention of impairments, disabilities and handicaps.

Development

Four dimensions (gross motor, fine motor and vision, hearing and speech, social).
Scales for development, applications and limitations.
Tests for special senses, applications and limitations.
'Screening for developmental delay', limitations.

Immunizations

Target group, contraindications.
Adverse reactions, interference with live vaccines and immunoglobulin, protective period.
Need for post-exposure vaccination, need for post-exposure chemoprophylaxis.
False contraindications (prematurity, atopic eczema, failure to thrive, suspected allergy to eggs, epilepsy, family history of epilepsy).

Aims of a consultation

Seven-task model:
1. To define the reasons for attendance.
2. To consider other problems.
3. To choose with the child and carers appropriate actions for each problem.
4. To achieve a shared understanding.
5. To involve the child and parents in the management plan.
6. To use time and resources appropriately.
7. To maintain good doctor–patient relationship.

Audit

The audit cycle.
Audit of structures, processes and outcomes.
Audit as quality assurance.
Audit as an educational activity.
Audit and evidence-based medicine.
Audit and resource allocation.

The long case

Bring along some colourful toys (for the distraction test), 1-inch (2.5 cm) cubes, 100s and 1000s, differently-coloured sweets, pencil and paper, a pair of blunt-headed scissors, measuring tape, stethoscope, ophthalmoscope, otoscope, small torch, tongue depressors, eye pads, ± paediatric tendon hammer, ± 512 Hz tuning fork.

Use the first minute to greet the mother and child. Make sure that they are comfortable. Their cooperation is of vital importance in the reliability and completeness of the history.

It is my habit to establish all the problems first, then go into the history of the individual problems in decreasing order of their significance, then ask for other histories.

The advantage of such an approach is that nothing important will be missed. You can have a heart attack if the mother suddenly voices out a history of epilepsy of the child when you have just 2 minutes left!

For each problem, ask the following:

1. When did it first present? How?
2. When was the diagnosis confirmed? How?
3. What are the exacerbating and relieving factors?
4. What immediate treatments have been given? What is the long-term plan of management?
5. What are the impacts of the problem? Does it affect growth, development, schooling, family life, financial situation, behaviour, etc.?
6. What medications is the child currently taking? (Dose, route, frequency, adverse effects, compliance?)

As soon as such information is obtained and clearly recorded, proceed to another problem. After finishing with all the problems, go through the following list quickly:

1. Age and occupations of parents.
2. Consanguinity
3. Pregnancy and complications.
4. Mode of delivery and complications.
5. Age and sex of siblings, general health of siblings.
6. Early problems (only if relevant).
7. The carers (e.g. grandparents, nursery).
8. Financial situation.
9. Immunization history ('up-to-date' is not enough, ask for specific vaccinations, e.g. influenza vaccine if asthmatic, pneumococcal vaccine if asplenic).
10. Developmental history (at least one example in each of the four areas, more examples if developmentally delayed).
11. Drug history, allergies.
12. Menstrual history if applicable.

At the physical examination, actively look for signs that might be present. Record significant negatives, e.g. absence of clubbing and central cyanosis for a child with congenital heart disease.

Always leave at least 5 to 10 minutes to organize the history and examination results. It is my habit to ask the child to draw himself, his family and a house (or copy simple shapes if younger) during that 5 to 10 minutes. The child can thus be distracted from disturbing you when you are organizing for the presentation. The finished artwork can also be presented to the examiners when relevant questions, e.g. development, family life, are asked.

Remember to document the growth parameters (height, weight and head circumference) and plot such on the percentile charts provided. Make sure that correct methods for measuring the height and the head circumference are used. (See the relevant MCQ questions later.)

Presenting the long case
There are generally three methods of presentation. The traditional method is to describe the most significant and recent problem and why the child was first admitted. As symptoms and signs are discussed first, the history is adjusted to sell the diagnosis to the examiners, thus demonstrating to the examiners that the candidate arrives at the diagnosis logically with the traditional symptom–sign–investigation approach.

However, this method may not be suitable if there are multiple important problems, as histories of the several problems will appear to be mixed up.

A second approach is to follow a strict chronological order. Thus, the history starts from the pregnancy, delivery and early problems to presentations of the recent problems.

This approach is clear in the time frame but will bore the examiners.

I would favour the problem-oriented approach. Thus, a short summarizing statement about all the important problems is given right at the start of the presentation. The individual problems will then be described in detail, stressing the symptoms and past investigation results which support the diagnoses. The birth, social, developmental, immunization and drug histories then follow.

This approach demonstrates that the candidate is not only regurgitating the story as told by the mother, but is presenting a processed account of problems faced by the child and the family, and using evidences to support the conclusions concomitantly.

For examination in the presence of the examiners, see the section on short cases below. An account of how to approach examiners' questions is found in the 'viva' section.

The short cases

Always greet and shake hands with the child and the carer before you examine the child. Listen carefully to the instructions. If you are asked to 'examine the heart,' this means the heart and not the cardiovascular system. Thus, do not waste time and irritate the examiners by feeling for radio-femoral delay. Relevant aspects of the general examination, e.g. looking for central cyanosis, are permissible.

Convince the examiners that you have done the examination several hundred times before. Aim not to pause after each step.

It is vital that your final diagnosis is supported by your clinical findings. If, for example, you describe a pansystolic murmur, it can only mean one of four things: ventricular septal defect (including A–V canal defects), mitral regurgitation, tricuspid regurgitation, or a poor candidate. Thus, if you do not think that the diagnosis is VSD, MR or TR, never describe a pansystolic murmur.

In other words, the final diagnosis is not as important as the processes by which you arrive at it. If you miss the diastolic phase of a continuous machinery murmur, describe such as a pansystolic murmur and diagnose a VSD instead of a PDA, marks will still be given. However, if you describe the murmur as pansystolic and diagnose a PDA, few or no marks are given, even though the final diagnosis is correct.

If you have no abnormal findings, say so. You may have been told to examine the heart of a child with atopic eczema.

Developmental examination

At least one short case is a developmental examination or an examination of the special senses.

If you are asked to perform a developmental examination, make sure that all four areas are covered with at least one examination of each area. You may ask for permission to pose questions to the mother.

For a hearing examination, the child is likely to be 6 to 18 months old, as the distraction test can then be performed. Ask for a noise detector to check for the background noise level. Be the distractor yourself and request the examiner to be the tester (sound-producer), not the other way round. Ask him to produce five different sounds (high, medium and low pitch sounds from a MEG warbler, human 'ss' and human 'hmmm') at 45° behind the child, so as not to give any hint of his presence by other sounds, shadows or odour.

Then, distract the child with a fast motion of the colourful toy, stop and catch the child's attention with a slow motion of the fingers. The tester gives the sound at the exact moment, the child turns and you have succeeded. Remember that the child has to turn at least twice on three attempts for each sound to pass the test.

Note that the history from the mother is more reliable than the distraction test. If allowed, ask some questions about the child's hearing and speech.

For the vision examination, the child is most likely to be more than 5 years old. Theoretically, single letter tests like STYCAR can be used from the age of 5. Snellen charts (better because of the crowding phenomenon) can be used from the age of 7.

Test at 6 m and not 3 m. Check for adequate lighting. Cover one eye with a pad and test for the corrected visual acuities (VAs) of the other eye. Express the VA in multiples of 1/60 (e.g. 24/60). Then examine the other eye. Test for uncorrected VA and near vision only if you have spare time.

If the largest letter cannot be read, try counting fingers. If this fails, shine a torch. Take a simple history from the mother if permitted.

Remember the definitions of 'blind' and 'partially sighted' (see the relevant MCQ question).

If a squint is obvious, ask the child to fixate on a moving object, thus determining whether it is a concomitant or inconcomitant (paralytic) squint. Perform the cover test for a concomitant squint to determine which is the dominant eye.

The viva

Dress up, speak up and shut up. Examiners usually expect 4–5 sentences to every question. Thus, answer in short, simple, relevant sentences. If you are content with your answer, the examiners will be too. Thus, shut up to wait for another question.

Some candidates use a tactic to guide the examiners to areas in which they are more knowledgeable. Experienced examiners see this easily and will not jump to the bait.

Some candidates save part of their knowledge in response to a question. Their theory is that, should a follow-up question be asked on the same subject, they will at least have something left to respond. However, this follow-up question may never come, and the examiners may think that the answer to the first question is incomplete.

Thus, answer clearly and relevantly. In answering simple, straightforward questions, do not imagine that the examiner knows everything and that you can add nothing more. Imagine that he knows nothing instead. Start from basic principles and imagine that you are teaching one of your patients on the subject. In this way, you will have more confidence to produce a well-organized, coherent response.

Objective Structured Clinical Examination (OSCE)

The OSCE, now part of the DCCH examination, is difficult to prepare for (for both the examiners and candidates alike) but easy to pass, provided that you know the inside tricks. Although some marks are given for the overall performance, most are given for specific tasks accomplished.

Thus, design 50 OSCE stations yourself and work out a marking scheme. When you arrive at the examination hall, this will become an automatic process. Demonstrate explicitly to the examiner that you know exactly which tasks score marks.

Introduction

The questions are likely to have been prepared months ago, and some are likely to be repeats of previous examinations. It is thus almost impossible to include stations with a child having acute signs or rare signs and therefore many of the children are normal. As the ability to reassure the parent is scorable, if no abnormal sign is detected, say boldly that the child is normal. Reassure the parent and repeat the statement that the child is normal (not 'may be' normal). In this way, the parent (examiner) must feel reassured (this is the rule of the game) and must give you marks.

The final advice

In the week immediately preceding the examination, spend 3 hours in your local medical library and review the most recent issues in paediatric journals. You will impress the examiners in your assessment of the long case, or during the viva, if one or two recent articles are quoted.

Best of luck in the DCH and other future examinations!

A A T Chuh

1 **The following sexually transmitted diseases are common in child sexual abuse:**

a) Lymphogranuloma venereum
b) Syphilis
c) Gonorrhoea
d) HIV infection
e) *Trichomonas vaginalis* infestation

2 **Preventive strategies for urinary tract infection include:**

a) Routine examination of the urine in pre-school examinations
b) Emptying the bladder regularly
c) Wiping from front to back for girls
d) Having a protocol to investigate all children with a proven urinary tract infection
e) Avoiding constipation

3 **Bruises are generally:**

a) Green or brown initially
b) Changing to blue or black in 2 or 3 days
c) Fading between 7 to 14 days
d) Resolving in 2 to 4 weeks
e) Of the same age when due to non-accidental injury

4 **A 6-month-old baby can:**

a) Pick up small objects between the finger and thumb
b) Pull himself to standing position
c) Play 'peek-a-boo' games
d) Stand holding on to furniture
e) Roll from prone to supine

5 **Measures to prevent accidental drug poisoning include:**

a) Never letting the child see an adult taking a drug
b) Keeping all syrups in tight fruit juice bottles
c) Telling the child that all medicines will be locked up
d) Not leaving medicines in the child's bedroom
e) Locking up all discarded medicines

6 **In examination of the cardiovascular system:**

a) A heart rate of 110/min at the age of 1 is normal
b) A heart rate of 135/min at the age of 4 is normal
c) A blood pressure of 85/55 at the age of 1 is normal
d) A blood pressure of 90/60 at the age of 3 is normal
e) The blood pressure should be checked as a screening procedure in the pre-school examination

7 Good prognostic factors in acute lymphoblastic leukaemia include:

a) Female sex
b) Normal haemoglobin value
c) Low initial white cell count
d) Low platelet count
e) Caucasian

8 The disability living allowance

a) Was previously represented by the Attendance allowance and the Mobility allowance
b) Is contributory
c) Has a care component and a mobility component
d) Will have the care component forfeited if the claimant lives in a publicly funded institute for 28 days or more
e) Is taxable

9 Secondary preventive strategies for hearing impairment include:

a) Genetic counselling
b) Rubella immunization for all children and women
c) Mumps immunization
d) Screening for hearing impairment
e) *Haemophilus influenzae* b vaccination for all children

10 A 3-year-old girl has recurrent episodes of bronchopneumonia with yellow-green sputum. The sputum is blood-stained. A chest X-ray shows evidence of bronchopneumonia with ring shadows involving bilateral lower lobes. The most likely diagnosis is:

a) A foreign body
b) Bronchiectasis
c) Recurrent aspiration
d) Tuberculosis
e) Extrinsic allergic alveolitis

11 A 3-year-old boy presents with acute ataxia. His urine is noted to have a sweet smell. On testing, valine, lecuine and isoleucine are present. The diagnosis is:

a) Homocystinuria
b) Cystinuria
c) Maple syrup urine disease
d) Cystinosis
e) Phenylketonuria

12 **Features of neurofibromatosis-1 include:**

a) Pheochromocytomata
b) Optic nerve gliomata
c) Retinal phakomata
d) Harmatomata
e) Duodenal carcinoids

13 **Seborrhoeic dermatitis:**

a) Is due to an abnormality of the sebaceous glands
b) Affects principally the intertrigenous areas
c) Affects the centre of the chest and the interscapular area
d) Affects the convexities of the face
e) Is treated by topical antifungal and steroid preparations

14 **The following statements are true:**

a) For children below 2 years, history and observation are adequate for the screening of non-disabling visual defects
b) Visual acuity should be routinely checked at 18 to 24 months
c) Visual acuity should be routinely checked at the time of school entry
d) Outreach services by orthoptists for pre-school children are cost-effective
e) Screening for dyslexia is currently recommended

15 **Members of the district handicap team include:**

a) Nurses
b) Psychologists
c) Community health doctors
d) Speech therapists
e) Teachers

16 **A 3-month-old baby can:**

a) Grasp objects voluntarily
b) Grasp his feet
c) Follow a dangling toy from one side to the other
d) Hold his bottle
e) Hold a rattle when placed in his hand

17 **Features of successful schools include:**

a) Positive atmosphere and ethos
b) Much parental involvement
c) High teacher expectation of pupils
d) Effective leadership
e) Teachers working and planning together

18   Complications of childhood obesity include:

a) Perthes' disease
b) Slipped femoral epiphyses
c) Blount's disease
d) Diabetes mellitus
e) Clumsiness

19   Common viral diseases causing photosensitivity include:

a) Rubella
b) Measles
c) Roseola infantum
d) Erythema infectiosum
e) Infectious mononucleosis

20   For exomphalos:

a) It is associated with gastrointestinal abnormalities
b) It is associated with genitourinary abnormalities
c) Surgical repair might relieve the respiratory embarrassment
d) A differential diagnosis is gastroschisis
e) A differential diagnosis is omphalocele

21   The following features are characteristic of congenital hypothyroidism:

a) Diarrhoea
b) Tachycardia
c) Hypertonia
d) Prolonged conjugated hyperbilirubinaemia
e) Umbilical hernia

22   A 7-month-old infant has become irritable, lasting for 6 hours. Bloodstained stools are passed twice. When examined he draws up his knees and screams. You should:

a) Set up an IV drip to correct the electrolyte imbalance
b) Prescribe a course of antibiotics
c) Refer him to a surgeon
d) Urgently check for amylase
e) Give suppositories to release the constipation

23   Signs of withdrawal in babies born to opiate-dependent mothers include:

a) Convulsions
b) Hypotonia
c) Constipation
d) Sweating
e) Fever

24 **The following statements are true:**

a) High protein, low salt diets are essential in nephrotic syndrome
b) Cushingoid features, due to steroids, are important in nephrotic syndrome
c) Anorexia is common in chronic renal failure
d) Low protein diet is helpful in acute renal failure
e) Protein accumulation is significant in children on dialysis

25 **Regarding the ECG:**

a) Hypokalaemia is associated with ST elevation
b) Hyperkalaemia is associated with the prolonged QT syndrome
c) Hypercalcaemia is associated with the prolonged QT syndrome
d) Hypocalcaemia is associated with shortened QT
e) A spreading of the QRST suggests hyperkalaemia

26 **Examples of X-linked recessive conditions are:**

a) Duchenne muscular dystrophy
b) Pseudohypoparathyroidism
c) G6PD deficiency
d) Haemophilia A
e) Haemophilia B

27 **The following therapeutic associations are true:**

a) Stevens–Johnson syndrome and steroids
b) Erythema nodosum and laser
c) Atopic eczema and emollients
d) Acrodermatitis enteropathica and vitamin E
e) Dermatitis herpetiformis and dapsone

28 **Causes of respiratory alkalosis include:**

a) Pneumonitis
b) Pulmonary oedema
c) Metabolic acidosis
d) Encephalitis
e) Fever

29 **An infant will:**

a) Look at your face at birth
b) Follow large objects to midline at birth
c) Follow large objects beyond midline at 3 months
d) Fixate on 100s and 1000s at 4 months
e) Take 100s and 1000s at 4 months

30 Molluscum contagiosum:

a) Is an adenovirus infection
b) Can be sexually transmitted
c) Presents as shiny, small papules with an umbilicated centre
d) Spontaneously recovers
e) Should be treated with cryosurgery for most cases in children

31 A child will not eat. Correct approaches to advise the mother include:

a) Give tonics
b) Absolutely no food between meals
c) Bribes
d) Punishment
e) Allow the child to choose the menu

32 The following statements are true:

a) Tics are repeated, purposeful movements resisted by the child
b) Gilles de la Tourette syndrome is the most severe form of tics
c) Haloperidol precipitates tics
d) Methylphenidate may be useful to treat tics
e) The parents can be asked to make the child deliberately repeat the movements

33 Wilson and Jungner's criteria for screening programmes include:

a) The test should be acceptable to the population
b) Only medical practitioners should be responsible for the testing
c) Treatment should be available
d) The test should be simple
e) The target group should be clearly defined

34 Causes of generalized lymphadenopathy include:

a) Glandular fever
b) Kawasaki disease
c) Still's disease
d) HIV infection
e) Phenobarbital

35 A 3-year-old boy has progressive proximal muscle weakness. He must climb up his knees to reach a standing position. Knee jerks are absent but ankle jerks appear normal. The most likely diagnosis is:

a) Myasthenia gravis
b) Duchenne muscular dystrophy
c) Dermatomyositis
d) Spinal muscular atrophy
e) Cerebral palsy

36 **Problems of babies born to mothers with poorly controlled diabetes mellitus include:**

a) Transposition of great vessels
b) Hyperglycaemia
c) Hypomagnesaemia
d) Shoulder dystocia
e) Anaemia

37 **An 18-month-old boy has pallor with haemoglobin 6.5 g/dL, reticulocytes 2% and blood film revealing hypochromacia with no spherocytes. His mother admitted feeding him with tea 'occasionally'. The most likely diagnosis is:**

a) Pernicious anaemia
b) Beta-thalassaemia major
c) Iron deficiency anaemia
d) G6PD deficiency
e) Aplastic anaemia

38 **In polyarthritis or polyarthralgia, the following are relevant:**

a) History of easy bruising
b) History of fever with macular rash on the first day of fever
c) That the child is on the Child Protection Register
d) History of recurrent abdominal pain with gastrointestinal bleeding
e) History of repeated self-mutilation

39 **A 2-year-old child with normal weight and height has 4–5 loose stools daily for 2 months. Corn and pieces of carrots are seen in the stool. The most likely diagnosis is:**

a) Cystic fibrosis
b) Toddler's diarrhoea
c) Munchausen syndrome by proxy
d) Malabsorption
e) Coeliac disease

40 **For congential rubella:**

a) The most susceptible period is the second trimester of pregnancy
b) Patent ductus arteriosus is an associated finding
c) Polycythaemia is commonly present
d) Scarring at angles of the mouth is characteristic
e) Immunoglobulins may be of use

41 **In hypercalcaemia:**

a) Wilson's disease is a cause
b) Williams' syndrome is a cause
c) Immobilization is a cause
d) Serum phosphate is normal in idiopathic hypercalcaemia
e) Serum phosphate is normal in hypervitaminosis D

42 **Common organisms causing neonatal pneumonia include:**

a) Group B haemolytic Streptococci
b) *Haemophilus influenzae*
c) *Escherichia coli*
d) *Mycoplasma pneumoniae*
e) *Chlamydia pneumoniae*

43 **Wilson and Jungner's criteria for screening programmes include the following:**

a) The test should be valid
b) The screening should be a continuous process, not once for-all
c) The cause of the condition should be clearly understood
d) Facilities for diagnosis and treatment should be available
e) The natural history of the condition should be known

44 **The following associations are true:**

a) Cisplatin and ototoxicity
b) Methotrexate and hepatotoxicity
c) Vincristine and haemorrhagic cystitis
d) Asparaginase and SIADH
e) Asparaginase and pancreatitis

45 **The main features of rickets in Asian children are:**

a) Renal disease
b) Vegetarian diet
c) Use of cows' milk for infant feeding
d) Anticonvulsants
e) Liver disease

46 **Contraindications to oral polio vaccine include:**

a) Frequent vomiting
b) History of encephalopathy
c) Another life vaccine received 2 months earlier
d) HIV infection
e) Leukaemia

47 **The following vaccines can be administered intradermally:**

a) Pneumococcal
b) BCG
c) Rabies
d) Typhoid
e) Meningococcal A+C

48 **A 16-year-old teenager presents with a left knee open wound contaminated with soil:**

a) Tetanus immunoglobin should be administered irrespective of the immunization history
b) If the immunization status is uncertain, a full 3 dose course of tetanus vaccine should be given
c) If the immunization status is uncertain, tetanus immunoglobulin should be given
d) If he has received a full 3 dose course and the last dose (or booster dose) was more than 10 years ago, a full 3 dose course of tetanus vaccine should be given
e) If the last dose (or booster dose) was within the last 10 years, 1 booster dose should be given

49 **The following statements regarding diphtheria are true:**

a) Diphtheria vaccine is a dead bacterial vaccine
b) Immunized children below 10 years with a contact history should receive one injection
c) Immunized children over 10 years with a contact history should receive one injection
d) Unimmunized children under 10 years with a contact history should receive three injections
e) Unimmunized contacts should receive a course of erythromycin or penicillin

50 **The following statements regarding 3-month colics are true:**

a) 3-month colics start at 3 to 4 months
b) They are most common at midnight
c) The infant usually draws up his legs
d) The cause is unknown
e) A change to soya formula is indicated

51 **Contraindications to oral polio vaccination include:**

a) Taking high-dose systemic steroids
b) High fever
c) Acute diarrhoea
d) Hypogammaglobulinaemia
e) Cerebral palsy

52 For diphtheria:

a) The Schick test should be performed in any 10-year-old child or over before diphtheria immunization
b) Diphtheria antitoxin should be given to suspected and confirmed cases of diphtheria
c) Diptheria antitoxin should be given to all unimmunized contacts
d) The dosage of diphtheria antitoxin for pharyngeal diphtheria is higher than that for nasal diphtheria
e) HIV carriers should receive the diphtheria vaccine

53 The following conditions should be routinely screened for all children:

a) Congenital haemoglobinopathies
b) Coeliac disease
c) Hypothyroidism
d) Lead poisoning
e) Vesicoureteric reflux

54 Language impairment is related to:

a) Gender
b) Laterality
c) Family size and birth order
d) Verbal interaction in the family
e) Social class

55 In asphyxia, features suggestive of primary apnoea include:

a) No response to stimulation
b) Gasping
c) Heart rate of 140/min
d) Heart rate of 76/min
e) Pale or greyish colour

56 Predisposing factors for iron deficiency include:

a) Infections
b) Hiatus hernia
c) Coeliac disease
d) Lead poisoning
e) Thalassaemia trait

57 Problems characteristic of a child with spina bifida include:

a) Kyphoscoliosis
b) Delayed puberty
c) Hydrocephalus
d) Incontinence
e) Elective mutism

58 **In Fallot tetralogy:**

a) Central cyanosis in the newborn period is characteristic
b) There is no murmur
c) A pansystolic murmur is characteristic
d) The heart looks normal on the chest X-ray
e) Cyanotic spells occur due to infundibular spasm

59 **Common problems of the small-for-date infant include:**

a) Hypoglycaemia
b) Infections
c) Hypothermia
d) Seizures
e) Polycythaemia

60 **In asphyxia, features suggestive of terminal apnoea include:**

a) Heart rate of 88/min and rising
b) Heart rate of 68/min, not rising
c) Pale or greyish colour
d) Grimacing to stimulation
e) Gasping

1   a) False   b) False   c) True   d) False   e) True

Chlamydia trachomatis serovars D-K may commonly cause genital infections in sex abuse cases. Such can be documented by culture or with PCR (polymerase chain reaction) or LCR (ligase chain reaction). Enzyme immunoassays are not accepted in court and serology is of limited use. LGV (lymphogranuloma venereum) is caused by *Chlamydia trachomatis* serovars L1–L3. It is mainly a tropical sexually transmitted infection and is rarely seen in developed countries. Syphilis is very rare in sex abuse cases. Most cases of infant and childhood HIV infection in developed countries are due to vertical transmission.

2   a) False   b) True   c) True   d) True   e) True

Routine urinalysis does not fulfil the criteria of a good screening test. Having a protocol is essential as a tertiary preventive strategy to prevent complications.

3   a) False   b) True   c) True   d) True   e) False

The colour of bruises shows much variation. However, bruises are generally red or purple initially. Excessive multiple bruises of different ages are suggestive of non-accidental injury.

4   a) False   b) False   c) True   d) False   e) True

Questions on development usually refer to the milestones reached by most children. Exceptions are the rule and the extent of parental and environmental stimulation is important. Most will develop a pincer grasp, and can pull themselves to the standing position at 9 months.

5   a) True   b) False   c) False   d) True   e) False

A child will imitate taking a drug if he sees an adult doing so. All medications should be kept in their original containers with the correct label and expiry date. Telling the child that medications will be locked up will stimulate him to find and unlock them. Discarded medication should be discarded, not locked up.

6   a) True   b) False   c) True   d) True   e) False

The heart rate is usually around 100/min at 4 years. Blood pressure measurement for all children does not fulfil the criteria as a good screening test at any age. The measurement should be taken only if clinically indicated.

7   a) True   b) False   c) True   d) False   e) True

A normal haemoglobin level and a low platelet count are poor prognostic factors.

8   a) True   b) False   c) True   d) True   e) False

The disability living allowance is non-contributory and non-means-tested. It is also tax free.

9   a) False   b) False   c) False   d) True   e) False

Genetic counselling is mainly for primary prevention, though sometimes secondary prevention may be achieved through case finding. Immunization against rubella, mumps and *Haemophilus influenzae* are examples of primary preventive strategies.

10   a) False   b) True   c) False   d) False   e) False

The grape-like shadows in the chest X-ray are very suggestive of bronchiectasis. The primary cause of the bronchiectasis cannot be identified from the information given.

11   a) False   b) False   c) True   d) False   e) False

12   a) True   b) True   c) False   d) False   e) True

Retinal phakomata and harmatomata of the internal organs are seen in tuberous sclerosis.

13   a) False   b) True   c) True   d) False   e) True

Seborrhoeic dermatitis has nothing to do with the sebaceous glands. The intertrigenous areas, i.e. neck, behind the ears, axillae, inguinal region and natal cleft, are principally affected. The concave surfaces of the face are typically involved. Involvement of the convexities of the face is characteristic of facial psoriasis, and, in adults, rosacea.

14   a) True   b) False   c) True   d) True   e) False

Checking the visual acuity at 18 to 24 months is difficult, unreliable and gives a low yield. It may even delay early treatment for cases missed, as parents are wrongly reassured. There is currently no instrument to screen for dyslexia which fulfils the criteria of a cost-effective screening test.

15   a) True   b) True   c) True   d) True   e) True

16   a) False   b) False   c) True   d) False   e) True

Most babies have voluntary grasp at 5 months. Most will grasp the feet and hold the bottle at least momentarily at 6 months.

17   a) True   b) True   c) True   d) True   e) True

18   a) True   b) True   c) True   d) True   e) True

Perthes' disease, slipped femoral epiphyses and Blount's disease are the three orthopaedic complications seen in childhood obesity. The risk of diabetes mellitus and hypertension is also increased in later life. Frequent chest infections is another common complication. Obese children may also be teased by other children, with psychological consequences.

19   a) **True**   b) **True**   c) **True**   d) **True**   e) **True**

20   a) **True**   b) **True**   c) **False**   d) **True**   e) **False**

Surgical repair might, in fact, increase the intra-abdominal pressure and exacerbate the respiratory distress. A gastroschisis has no skin covering. It is most commonly to the right inferior aspect of the umbilicus. Omphalocele is another name for exomphalos.

21   a) **False**   b) **False**   c) **False**   d) **False**   e) **True**

Constipation, bradycardia, hypotension and prolonged unconjugated hyperbilirubinaemia are characteristic of congenital hypothyroidism.

22   a) **True**   b) **False**   c) **True**   d) **False**   e) **False**

The history is very suggestive of intussusception, a paediatric emergency not to be missed. When examined, a sausage-shaped mass may be palpable in the right *upper* quadrant of the abdomen. The stool is like redcurrant jelly. Hydrostatic reduction will be attempted by the surgeon, failure of which necessitates laparotomy for reduction and resection of the segment if needed.

23   a) **True**   b) **False**   c) **False**   d) **True**   e) **True**

The manifestations are like those in adults. The baby is irritable. Hypotonia is not a feature. Diarrhoea is characteristic, not constipation.

24   a) **False**   b) **True**   c) **True**   d) **True**   e) **False**

High protein, low salt diets are not palatable. The benefits are uncertain and, as steroids are effective for most cases, such diets are not currently recommended. Cushingoid effects are common and important. Thus, healthy eating should be emphasized. For children on dialysis, protein loss is significant, not accumulation.

25   a) **False**   b) **False**   c) **False**   d) **False**   e) **True**

Hypokalaemia leads to ST depression. Both hypokalaemia and hypocalcaemia are associated with the prolonged QT syndrome.

26   a) **True**   b) **False**   c) **True**   d) **True**   e) **True**

Pseudohypoparathyroidism is one of the few conditions which are X-linked dominant.

27   a) **True**   b) **False**   c) **True**   d) **False**   e) **True**

The associated cause of erythema nodosum should be identified and treated. Otherwise, only symptomatic treatment for the local lesion is necessary. Acrodermatitis enteropathica is related to zinc deficiency. Vitamin E is not implicated.

| 28 | a) True | b) True | c) True | d) True | e) True |

| 29 | a) True | b) False | c) True | d) False | e) False |

An infant will follow objects to the midline at 1 to 2 months, fixate on 100s and 1000s at 5 to 6 months and attempt to take 100s and 1000s at 6 to 8 months, though there is much variation.

| 30 | a) False | b) True | c) True | d) True | e) False |

Molluscum contagiosum is caused by a pox virus. It is not commonly realized that it can be sexually transmitted. The morphological description is classical for the lesion. However, diagnosis without investigations can be difficult when lesions are few and the umbilication is not seen. Spontaneous recovery is the rule. However, the process might take more than 1 to 2 years. Chemical ablation or cryosurgery may be indicated for adults for cosmetic reasons. For small children, no active treatment is indicated.

| 31 | a) False | b) True | c) False | d) False | e) False |

No food between meals and non-encouragement of food fads are central in the management of food refusal. Such rules are much more easily said than done. It must be realized that the family as a whole should be managed, as the 'pathology' does not lie with the child alone.

| 32 | a) False | b) True | c) False | d) False | e) True |

The movements in tics serve no purpose. Haloperidol might control tics. Methylphenidate, used in the management of hyperkinetic disorder, might precipitate tics in some children. Some cases respond to repeated, deliberate movements as a behavioural aversion therapy.

| 33 | a) True | b) False | c) True | d) True | e) True |

Such criteria are central to the development and assessment of screening procedures in child health promotion programmes. A team approach is encouraged and other health professionals, such as health visitors and district and practice nurses, are essential in the provision of such services.

| 34 | a) True | b) False | c) True | d) True | e) False |

The lymphadenopathy associated with Kawasaki disease is non-suppurative and is mainly localized in the cervical region. It is phenytoin which can cause lymphadenopathies.

| 35 | a) False | b) True | c) False | d) False | e) False |

Note that dermatomyositis can also present as proximal muscle weakness. However, the absence of dermatological signs makes Duchenne muscular dystrophy the most likely diagnosis.

36	**a) True**	**b) False**	**c) True**	**d) True**	**e) False**

Hypoglycaemia may be present rather than hyperglycaemia. Polycythaemia is likely rather than anaemia. Erb's palsy in such infants is related to the shoulder dystocia.

37	**a) False**	**b) False**	**c) True**	**d) False**	**e) False**

38	**a) True**	**b) True**	**c) True**	**d) True**	**e) True**

In haemophilia, there is easy bruising. Rubella presents with fever and macular rash on the first day of fever. Arthralgia, thrombocytopenia and encephalitis are possible complications of rubella. Non-accidental injuries may lead to multiple fracture. A child with inflammatory bowel diseases will have recurrent abdominal pain with gastrointestinal bleeding. Repeated self-mutilation is characteristic of Lesch–Nyhan syndrome. HGPRT is deficient leading to hyperuricaemia.

39	**a) False**	**b) True**	**c) False**	**d) False**	**e) False**

Toddler's diarrhoea is common and some regard it as the paediatric equivalent of adult irritable bowel syndrome. No treatment other than reassurance is needed.

40	**a) False**	**b) True**	**c) False**	**d) False**	**e) True**

The most susceptible period is the first trimester. Thus serial measurements of IgG and IgM titres are essential if rubella or contact history is suspected. Anaemia may be present in the infant. Rhagades are scarring at the angles of the mouth, characteristic of congenital syphilis. Immunoglobulins may be of value for women with confirmed rubella infection in the first trimester who would not consider termination of pregnancy. The extent of fetal damage may be decreased.

41	**a) False**	**b) True**	**c) True**	**d) True**	**e) True**

Cirrhosis in Wilson's disease may lead to hypocalcaemia but not hypercalcaemia. William's syndrome is idiopathic hypercalcaemia of infancy.

42	**a) True**	**b) False**	**c) True**	**d) False**	**e) False**

43	**a) True**	**b) True**	**c) False**	**d) True**	**e) True**

The course but not the cause of the condition should be fairly well understood before screening can be justified.

44	**a) True**	**b) True**	**c) False**	**d) False**	**e) True**

It is cyclophosphamide which leads to haemorrhagic cystitis. Vincristine is one of the causes of inappropriate antidiuretic hormone secretion.

45	**a) False**	**b) True**	**c) True**	**d) False**	**e) False**

46	a) True	b) False	c) False	d) False	e) True

Oral polio vaccination should be postponed if the child has high fever, diarrhoea or vomiting. A system must be present so as to call back the defaulters. Two live vaccines should either be administered on the same day to different sites on the body, or be separated by at least 3 weeks. HIV infection and AIDS are not contraindications to the oral polio vaccine, although the physician or the paediatrician may, at his choice, offer inactivated polio vaccine instead of oral polio. An immunocompromised state such as leukaemia is a contraindication for oral polio vaccine.

47	a) False	b) True	c) True	d) True	e) False

Most vaccines, including the pneumococcal and meningococcal A+C vaccines, are given either by the intramuscular or deep subcutaneous routes. The only method of administration for BCG is intradermal. Rabies can be given by intradermal, intramuscular or deep subcutaneous routes. For typhoid, the first dose must be given by intramuscular or deep subcutaneous route while subsequent doses can also be given intradermally.

48	a) True	b) True	c) True	d) False	e) False

If a full 3-dose course was already given and the last dose (or booster dose) was more than 10 years ago, 1 booster dose only should be given. As this is a high-risk wound, tetanus immunoglobulin should be administered concomitantly. If the last dose of a 3-dose course (or booster dose) was within the recent 10 years, vaccination is not indicated provided that the history of vaccination is reliable, preferably with written proof. In view of the high-risk wound, tetanus immunoglobulin is to be given.

49	a) False	b) True	c) True	d) True	e) True

Diphtheria vaccine is a toxoid. For immunized children over 10 years with a contact history, 1 low-dose injection is given. For unimmunized children under 10 years with contact history, three injections are given at monthly intervals. Irrespective of immunization, unimmunized contacts should be given erythromycin or penicillin. The Schick test is no longer available. The decision to give diphtheria vaccine does not depend on the test result any more.

50	a) False	b) False	c) True	d) True	e) False

Three-month colics typically cease at 3 to 4 months. They are most common in the evening. Though many theories have been proposed, the cause is still unknown. Virtually all cases resolve spontaneously. No treatment is indicated.

51	a) True	b) True	c) True	d) True	e) False

High-dose systemic steroids may lead to immunosuppression and are thus a contraindication. Prophylactic inhaled steroids for asthma and replacement steroids are, however, not contraindications to the oral polio vaccine. Vaccination should be postponed if the child has high fever, vomiting or diarrhoea.

17

52   a) False   b) True   c) False   d) True   e) True

Materials for the Schick test are no longer available. The decision to give diphtheria vaccine does not depend on the test result. For unimmunized contacts, a course of three injections of vaccine is given, together with a course of erythromycin or penicillin.

53   a) False   b) False   c) True   d) False   e) False

Screening for congenital haemoglobinopathies is only justifiable in certain districts where the proportion of ethnic minorities is high. Routine screening for coeliac disease, lead poisoning and vesicoureteric reflux does not fulfil the criteria of cost-effective screening tests.

54   a) True   b) False   c) True   d) True   e) True

Male children are much more commonly affected by language impairment. Laterality is of no relevance. The only child and the first-born child in the family are the least likely to have language difficulties.

55   a) False   b) True   c) True   d) False   e) False

No response to stimulation, a non-rising heart rate of less than 100/min and pale or greyish colour all suggest terminal apnoea.

56   a) True   b) True   c) True   d) True   e) False

57   a) True   b) False   c) True   d) True   e) False

Children with spina bifida might have premature puberty. They also have 'cocktail party speech' instead of mutism.

58   a) False   b) False   c) False   d) False   e) True

Central cyanosis is present only if there is reversal of shunt or when there are cyanotic spells due to infundibular spasms. Whilst there is no murmur for the high VSD, a pulmonary stenosis murmur is present. It is an ejection systolic murmur in the pulmonary area not radiating to the neck. The heart is characteristically boot-shaped on the chest X-ray.

59   a) True   b) True   c) True   d) True   e) True

The seizures are commonly due to hypoglycaemia, hypoxia or hypocalcaemia.

60   a) False   b) True   c) True   d) False   e) False

A rising heart rate, even if less than 100/min, suggests primary apnoea. A non-rising heart rate less than 100/min suggests terminal apnoea. Grimacing as a reaction to stimulation and gasping are features of primary apnoea.

61 **The following are appropriate dosages for children:**

a) Erythromycin 250 mg/kg/24 h orally
b) Paraldehyde 0.2 ml/kg per dose intramuscularly
c) Phenobarbital 100 mg/kg/24 h orally
d) Carbamazepine 100 mg/kg/24 h orally
e) Sodium valproate 100 mg/kg/24 h orally

62 **Major causes of neonatal mortality include:**

a) Immaturity
b) Neonatal jaundice
c) Respiratory distress syndrome
d) Infection
e) Haemorrhagic disease of the newborn

63 **Examples of primary preventive activities include:**

a) Accident prevention
b) Immunization
c) Prevention of child abuse
d) Prevention of complications in accidental injuries
e) Health education

64 **Assessment of an obese child can include:**

a) Diet history
b) Chromosomal analysis
c) Body mass index
d) Thyroid function tests
e) Skinfold thickness

65 **The following are compatible with Klinefelter's syndrome:**

a) Long legs
b) Small testes
c) Attending normal schools
d) Absence of gynaecomastia
e) 47 XYY

66 **When measuring the head circumference of an infant:**

a) A rigid ruler is advisable
b) A paper or linen tape is advisable
c) The external occipital protuberance should be used as a reference point
d) The largest circumference passing through the reference point is taken
e) Moulding and oedema should be clearly recorded

67   The following approaches may assist a child with vision problems:

a) Magnifiers
b) Tactile maps
c) Learn Braille
d) Tape recording
e) Typewriting

68   In cystic fibrosis:

a) Regular physiotherapy is essential
b) Nebulized bronchodilators may be of benefit
c) Early, long-term use of nebulized antibiotics is advocated
d) Regular vigorous exercise should be encouraged
e) Supply of donors is limited for heart/lung transplantation

69   The following statements about milk banks are true:

a) Boiling is advised for sterilization
b) Breast milk from milk banks can prevent necrotizing enterocolitis
c) Strict screening for milk donors is vital
d) The number of milk banks is increasing as mothers are becoming more aware of the benefits of breast milk
e) The use of milk banks should be especially encouraged for preterm babies

70   Causes of conjugated neonatal hyperbilirubinaemia include:

a) Biliary atresia
b) Spherocytosis
c) Cystic fibrosis
d) Alagille's syndrome
e) Congenital rubella

71   Neonatal myasthenia gravis:

a) Occurs in 50% of all infants born by mothers with myasthenia gravis
b) Has a delayed onset of symptoms
c) Is usually confirmed by symptomatic improvement after intravenous edrophonium
d) Is treated with the anticholinergic drug neostigmine
e) Has a guarded prognosis

72   In cerebral palsy, the following phenomena make feeding difficult:

a) Postural problems
b) Swallowing problems
c) Hypotonia
d) Chewing problems
e) Reflux

73 Characteristic features of achondroplasia include:

a) Wide and flattened nose bridge
b) Large head
c) Lumbar lordosis
d) Trident hands
e) Mild mental retardation

74 In tubotympanic disease:

a) Poor personal hygiene is implicated as a factor
b) Frequent upper respiratory tract infection is associated
c) A clear discharge is characteristic
d) Hearing impairment is associated
e) Surgical approach to close the tympanic perforation is usually indicated

75 With regard to the ECG:

a) The normal range of axis in a newborn is +120° to −170°
b) Right axis deviation is characteristic for ASD primum
c) Left axis deviation is usual in Fallot's tetralogy
d) Right axis deviation is usual in tricuspid atresia
e) Dextrocardia leads to inverted P-wave in lead I

76 Characteristic features in lead poisoning include:

a) Basophilic stripping of red blood cells
b) An abnormally low blood lead level
c) Lead lines at the end of long bones
d) Lead particles in the bowel shown on the X-ray
e) A low, free erythrocyte protoporphyrin level

77 Causes of true precocious puberty include:

a) Intracranial tumours
b) Congenital adrenal hyperplasia
c) Familial
d) Gonodal tumours
e) Cranial radiotherapy

78 An 18-month-old child presents with an abdominal mass crossing the midline. CT shows a calcified mass with two normal kidneys. The likely diagnosis is:

a) Nephroblastoma
b) Hepatoblastoma
c) Neuroblastoma
d) Hodgkin's lymphoma
e) Non-Hodgkin's lymphoma

79 **In scabies:**

a) The faces of babies are characteristically spared
b) The diagnosis must be confirmed before treatment
c) The whole family must be treated together
d) Benzyl benzoate should be applied
e) The child should be re-treated if the pruritus persists 2 weeks after standard treatment

80 **The following statements are true:**

a) Secondary enuresis means enuresis with an identified secondary cause
b) Mental retardation is a common cause of primary enuresis
c) Enuresis is regarded as a specific developmental delay if no secondary cause is identifiable
d) Sexual abuse should be suspected as a cause of enuresis only if convincing evidence is present
e) Epilepsy is an uncommon cause of enuresis

81 **A medical adviser in adoption:**

a) Should direct the adoption agency to obtain health information of the natural parents and prospective adopters and health and developmental information of the child
b) Should have a good knowledge of the medical network in order to gather information
c) Should try to make an accurate prediction of the future development of the child
d) Should have good communication skills
e) Should be ready to liaise with other professional colleagues

82 **The following conditions are autosomal dominant:**

a) Hunter's syndrome
b) 21-hydroxylase deficiency
c) Myotonic dystrophy
d) Beta thalassaemia
e) Alpha-1-antitrypsin deficiency

83 **The following associations are correct:**

a) Plain abdominal X-ray and radio-opaque stones
b) DMSA scan and renal scarring
c) DTPA scan and function of different parts of the kidneys
d) Ultrasound and vesicoureteric reflux
e) Micturating cystourethrogram and vesicoureteric reflux

84 **Causes of napkin rash include:**

a) Irritant contact dermatitis
b) Psoriasis
c) Seborrhoeic dermatitis
d) Candidiasis
e) Histiocytosis X

85 **Interpretation of the Heaf test:**

a) Grade 0 – no induration at the puncture sites
b) Grade 1 – discrete induration at 2 or more sites
c) Grade 2 – induration sites merge with one another
d) Grade 3 – the centre of the ring is also indurated. The entire indurated site becomes 10–20 mm wide
e) Grade 4 – the indurated site becomes over 20 mm wide. Vesiculation or ulceration may be present

86 **Characteristic features of the African variant of G6PD deficiency include:**

a) Haemoglobin often below 6 g/dl
b) Short, latent period of haemolysis after exposure
c) Females commonly affected
d) Self limiting haemolysis
e) Favism

87 **A 2-year-old girl has a large abdominal mass. CT shows the mass attached to an abnormal-looking kidney. Associated findings include:**

a) Haematuria
b) Calcification seen on the abdominal X-ray
c) Hemihypertrophy
d) Abnormal chest X-ray
e) Elevated urine catecholamines

88 **Interpretation of the Mantoux test:**

a) The result should be read 24–48 hours later
b) Induration of 2 mm: negative
c) Induration of 9 mm: negative
d) Induration of 14 mm: positive, consider chemoprophylaxis
e) Induration of 20 mm: positive, consider chemoprophylaxis

89 The following are appropriate dosage for children:

a) Paracetamol 10 mg/kg/24 h orally
b) Amoxycillin 200 mg/kg/24 h orally
c) Erythromycin 50 mg/kg/24 h orally
d) Cephalexin 50 mg/kg/24 h orally
e) Phenobarbital 5 mg/kg/24 h intramuscularly

90 Equipment needed in a Child Health Clinic includes:

a) Sound level meter
b) Tympanometer
c) Spoon-and-cup
d) *MEG* warbler
e) Visual acuity charts

91 The following associations are true:

a) Lead poisoning and punctate basophilia
b) Post-splenectomy and Heinz bodies
c) G6PD deficiency and Heinz bodies
d) Thalassaemia and target cells
e) Iron deficiency anaemia and target cells

92 Congenital rubella infection can lead to:

a) Hearing impairment
b) Cataracts
c) Microcephaly
d) Cerebral calcification
e) Heart defects

93 The following associations are true:

a) Gaucher's disease and hepatosplenomegaly
b) Hurler syndrome and hyperacusis
c) Wilson's disease and self-mutilation
d) Tay–Sachs disease and a red cherry spot on the macula
e) Phenylketonuria and corneal opacity

94 X-linked dominant disorders include:

a) Incontinentia pigmentiae
b) Rett's syndrome
c) Pseudohypoparathyroidism
d) Haemophilia C
e) Hypochondroplasia

95 **The following features support a diagnosis of depression:**

a) Increased appetite
b) Difficulty in falling asleep
c) Putting on weight
d) Early morning wakening
e) Feeling of worthlessness

96 **In pertussis:**

a) Conjuctival haemorrhages are common
b) The inspiratory whoop is always present
c) Death is usually due to pneumothorax
d) Antibiotics modify the course of the disease
e) The yield of isolating *Bordetella pertussis* is higher in the paroxysmal phase than in the catarrhal phase

97 **The following conditions are compatible with a paralytic squint:**

a) Cranial nerve agenesis
b) Inherited failure of fusion of images
c) Cataracts
d) Refractive errors
e) Raised intracranial pressure

98 **Risk factors for neonates with hearing impairment include:**

a) Congenital rubella infection
b) Breast milk jaundice
c) Family history of hearing impairment
d) Congenital toxoplasma infection
e) Malformation of pinnae

99 **Signs of emotional abuse and neglect include:**

a) Frozen watchfulness
b) Organic failure to thrive
c) Laser gaze
d) Deprivation dwarfism
e) Deprivation hands and feet

100 **Causes of tall stature are:**

a) Hyperparathyroidism
b) Hypoparathyroidism
c) Hypothyroidism
d) Hyperthyroidism
e) Congenital adrenal hyperplasia

101 The following medications should be avoided during breast feeding:

a) Nitrazepam
b) Ergot derivatives
c) Nalidixic acid
d) Naproxen
e) Paracetamol

102 A child with haemophilia A:

a) Will bleed only after severe trauma if the factor VIII level is 50 units/dl
b) Will have spontaneous bleeding if the factor VIII level is 15 units/dl
c) Should safely be prescribed with narcotics for joint pain
d) Has normal bleeding time
e) Has normal activated partial thromboplastin time

103 The following are true associations:

a) Neurofibromatosis-2 and autosomal dominance
b) Sturge-Weber syndrome and autosomal recessiveness
c) Ataxia-telangiectasia and X-linked recessiveness
d) Tuberous sclerosis and autosomal dominance
e) Ectodermal dysplasia and autosomal recessiveness

104 The following vaccines are given by intramuscular or deep subcutaneous route:

a) DPT
b) BCG
c) MMR
d) *Haemophilus influenzae* b
e) Meningococcal A+C

105 The height of a 3-year-old girl is below the –3 SD curve. Her parents are tall. Initial investigations include:

a) X-ray of left hand and wrist
b) X-ray of legs and feet
c) Blood picture
d) Erythrocyte sedimentary rate
e) Thyroid function tests

106 In patent ductus arteriosus:

a) A continuous machinery murmur is characteristic
b) The pulse is often weak
c) A weak apical impulse is usual
d) Left ventricular hypertrophy is usually seen on the ECG
e) The risk of bacterial endocarditis is not significantly increased

107 **Duties of the health visitor might include:**

a) Surveillance of children at risk of abuse
b) Supervision of children in care
c) Ear syringing
d) Visiting all children under 5 years
e) Mobilization of resources in the community

108 **With regard to the APGAR score:**

a) 2 points are given for a pulse of 88/min
b) 1 point is given for irregular gasps
c) An initially satisfactory score guarantees an uneventful perinatal period
d) A score of 2 at 10 minutes carries a worse prognosis than a score of 2 at 5 minutes
e) The lowest possible score is 1

109 **For the court orders:**

a) The Emergency Protection Order can be applied by anyone
b) A residence order defines with whom the child is to live
c) A contact order confers parental responsibility
d) A care order lasts until the child is 18 years of age
e) A supervision order lasts until the child is 16 years of age

110 **Recommendations to prevent iron deficiency include:**

a) Not giving tea to young children
b) Iron supplements to children with thalassaemia
c) Iron supplements for premature infants
d) The early introduction of cows' milk
e) Weaning to mixed feeding at 6 months of age

111 **Duties of the health visitor might include:**

a) Education for mothers in the child health clinics
b) Wound management
c) Immunization
d) Screening for hearing impairments
e) Measuring the growth parameters

112 **A 5-month-old girl of Far Eastern origin develops a hypochromic microcytic anaemia with target cells. Hb F and Hb A_2 are increased with no Hb A present. The diagnosis is:**

a) Sickle cell disease
b) Beta thalassaemia trait
c) Beta thalassaemia major
d) Spherocytosis
e) Pyruvate kinase deficiency

113 **With regard to behavioural disturbances:**

a) Barbiturates may cause aggressiveness
b) Methylphenidate may cause over-activity
c) Theophylline may cause over-activity
d) Amphetamine may cause excited behaviour
e) Ephedrine may cause irritability

114 **The following medications should be avoided during breastfeeding:**

a) Trimethoprim
b) Metformin
c) Digoxin
d) Salicylates
e) Tetracycline

115 **An 18-month-old child has bloody diarrhoea with high fever for 2 days. The likely causal organisms may be:**

a) Shigella
b) Adenovirus
c) Rotavirus
d) Hepatitis A
e) Campylobacter

116 **Indications for circumcision are:**

a) Most of the other boys in the class have been circumcized
b) Recurrent paraphimosis
c) Frequent masturbation
d) Family history of carcinoma of the penis
e) Neglected nappy rash leading to scarring

117 **Risk factors for children with hearing impairment include:**

a) Cleft palate
b) Recurrent otitis media
c) History of meningitis
d) Parental suspicion of hearing impairment
e) Cerebral palsy

118 **Characteristic findings in a preterm baby include:**

a) Rounded back when held sitting
b) Hand reaches beyond tip of shoulder
c) Incomplete wrist flexion
d) Legs not flat on couch when lying supine
e) High pelvis when lying prone

119 **The following associations are true:**

a) Biceps reflex: C5 C6
b) Knee jerk: L2 L3
c) Ankle jerk: S2 S3
d) Cremasteric reflex: L3 L4
e) Triceps reflex: C7 C8

120 **Bleeding time is increased in:**

a) Factor VIII deficiency
b) Factor IX deficiency
c) Von Willebrand's disease
d) Factor X deficiency
e) Factor XI deficiency

61 a) **False**   b) **True**   c) **False**   d) **False**   e) **False**

The commonly used dosages are: erythromycin 50 mg/kg/24 h orally, phenobarbital 5 mg/kg/24 h orally, carbamazepine 10–20 mg/kg/24 h orally and sodium valproate 20–30 mg/kg/24 h orally.

62 a) **True**   b) **False**   c) **True**   d) **True**   e) **False**

Other major causes of neonatal mortality are asphyxia, birth injury and congenital abnormalities.

63 a) **True**   b) **True**   c) **True**   d) **False**   e) **True**

The prevention of complications is tertiary prevention. Disabilities and handicaps are decreased in number and severity. Health education is mostly for primary prevention, though opportunities exist to assist early detection to some extent, i.e. secondary prevention.

64 a) **True**   b) **True**   c) **True**   d) **True**   e) **True**

Chromosomal analysis may reveal, say, trisomy 21. Thyroid function tests might detect hypothyroidism.

65 a) **True**   b) **True**   c) **True**   d) **True**   e) **False**

Learning difficulties are usually mild for children and adolescents with Klinefelter's syndrome. Gynaecomastia is not necessarily present to make the diagnosis. It is 47 XXY rather than 47 XYY which is related.

66 a) **False**   b) **False**   c) **True**   d) **True**   e) **True**

A narrow metal tape should best be used. The external occipital protuberance is the occiput. With this as the reference point, three measurements are taken for the occipital-frontal circumference. The largest, not the average, of the three is taken to be the head circumference. Any moulding or oedema or cephalhaematoma should be clearly recorded, and the measurement should be repeated several days later.

67 a) **True**   b) **True**   c) **True**   d) **True**   e) **True**

68 a) **True**   b) **True**   c) **False**   d) **True**   e) **True**

In most children with cystic fibrosis, the airway obstruction has a reversible component. Thus, nebulized bronchodilators might be of benefit. The policies for long-term antibiotics vary in different centres. However, most would agree that long-term antibiotics, systemic or localized, should be reserved for those with more advanced disease. The use of DNase may improve the lung function for some children and adolescents with cystic fibrosis.

69   a) False   b) True   c) True   d) False   e) True

Boiling destroys IgA and thus a major advantage of breast milk disappears. Strict screening for donors hopes to prevent infections such as HIV. Although mothers are becoming more aware of the benefits of breast milk, they are even more aware of the possibility of HIV transmission. Thus the number of milk banks is decreasing.

70   a) True   b) False   c) True   d) True   e) True

71   a) False   b) False   c) True   d) False   e) False

Only 10 to 15% of the infants born to mothers with myasthenia gravis (MG) will develop neonatal MG. The symptoms usually appear in the first 24 hours. Neostigmine is a cholinesterase inhibitor, not an anticholinergic agent. The prognosis is excellent for those with no other congenital abnormalities.

72   a) True   b) True   c) False   d) True   e) True

Hypertonia is an obstacle, not hypotonia.

73   a) True   b) True   c) True   d) True   e) False

Intelligence is characteristically not affected in achondroplasia and hypochondroplasia.

74   a) True   b) True   c) False   d) True   e) False

Poor personal hygiene, poor social backgrounds and repeated upper respiratory tract infections (URIs) are risk factors for tubotympanic disease. The discharge is usually purulent or mucopurulent. A medical approach to treat the URIs is indicated.

75   a) True   b) False   c) False   d) False   e) True

Left axis deviation is characteristic for tricuspid atresia, with negative QRS in I and aV_F. In dextrocardia, the P-wave is inverted in I and aV_R and upright in III.

76   a) True   b) False   c) True   d) True   e) False

The lead level in the blood is elevated. The free erythrocyte protoporphyrin level is high.

77   a) True   b) False   c) True   d) False   e) True

'True' precocious puberty means that the hypothalamic-pituitary-adrenal axis is involved.

78   a) False   b) False   c) True   d) False   e) False

79   **a) False**   **b) False**   **c) True**   **d) False**   **e) False**

Unlike adults, the faces of infants are characteristically affected. It is, of course, best to identify the mite in the burrows before treatment. This is, however, not always possible. A contact history with characteristic findings is a good justification to start treatment. The failure to insist that the whole family should be treated together is *the* commonest cause for failure of eradication. Benzyl benzoate is too much of an irritant to be used in infants. Malathion can be used instead. The pruritus in scabies is due to sensitization. It will persist for 4 to 6 weeks after successful eradication. Unnecessary re-treatment courses will lead to irritant contact dermatitis and resistance. A sedating antihistamine should be given at night to reduce the itching.

80   **a) False**   **b) True**   **c) True**   **d) False**   **e) True**

Primary enuresis is enuresis without a preceding period of continence. Secondary enuresis (onset enuresis) is enuresis occurring after a period of normal urinary habit. There is a higher probability of identifying a secondary cause in secondary enuresis. Enuresis with no cause identified possesses many characteristics shared by other types of specific developmental delay. A high index of suspicion is required to diagnose sexual abuse and evidence should be actively sought.

81   **a) True**   **b) True**   **c) False**   **d) True**   **e) True**

The medical adviser should impress upon the potential adopters that early developmental assessment does not have a high predictability.

82   **a) False**   **b) False**   **c) True**   **d) False**   **e) False**

Hunter's syndrome is X-linked recessive while all the other types of mucopolysaccharidosis are autosomal recessive. Congenital adrenal hyperplasia due to absent or decreased 21-hydroxylase and betathalassaemia are autosomal recessive. Alpha-1-antitripsin deficiency is best described as autosomal co-dominant. The normal phenotype of the protease inhibitor system is PiMM. PiZZ is most related with liver disease. PiMS, PiMZ and PiSZ are intermediate forms. Pi null/null is associated with early adult-onset chest disease (emphysemia) but no liver disease. Myotonic dystrophy is a maternally-transmitted autosomal dominant disease with triplet repeat expansion, with phenomena of 'imprinting' and 'anticipation' (see standard textbooks for details).

83   **a) True**   **b) True**   **c) True**   **d) False**   **e) True**

Ultrasound cannot accurately detect reflux.

84   **a) True**   **b) True**   **c) True**   **d) True**   **e) True**

Irritant contact dermatitis is the common chemical dermatitis. Candidiasis usually accompanies a pre-existing chemical dermatitis or follows oral antibiotics.

85   **a) True**   **b) False**   **c) True**   **d) False**   **e) False**

In grade 1, there are discrete indurations in four or more sites. In grade 2, the six spots of induration merge with each other, thus forming a complete circle with a clear centre. In grade 3, the centre of the circle is also indurated and the entire indurated site becomes 5 to 10 mm wide. In grade 4, the indurated site is over 10 mm wide. Vesiculation or ulceration may be present.

86   a) False   b) False   c) True   d) True   e) False

Very low haemoglobin values and favism are characteristic features of the Mediterranean variant of G6PD deficiency. The African variant has a long (24–36 h) latent period between exposure and haemolysis while the Mediterranean variant has a short (3–24 h) latent period.

87   a) True   b) False   c) True   d) True   e) False

Calcifications seen on the abdominal X-ray and elevated urine catecholamines are characteristic features of neuroblastoma. The abnormal chest X-ray is due to metastases of the nephroblastoma.

88   a) False   b) True   c) False   d) False   e) True

The result of the Mantoux test should be read at 48 to 72 hours. An induration of 0–4 mm is negative and corresponds to Heaf grades 0 and 1. Induration of 5–14 mm is positive, corresponding to Heaf grade 2. For such a result, no further action is necessary if the test is done as routine screening. An induration of 15 mm or larger is positive, corresponding to Heaf grades 3 and 4. Referral to a chest clinic should be considered and chemoprophylaxis might be needed in some cases.

89   a) False   b) False   c) True   d) True   e) True

The usual dosage of paracetamol is 75 mg/kg/24 h orally. That of amoxycillin is 25–50 mg/kg/24 h orally.

90   a) True   b) False   c) False   d) True   e) True

A tympanometer should be equipped in an audiology clinic. Spoon-and-cup is now not recommended as a suitable sound source for the distraction test. A soft high-pitch 's', a soft low-pitch humming, and a low, medium and high pitch sound from a MEG warbler should be used.

91   a) True   b) False   c) True   d) True   e) True

Howell–Jolly bodies are seen in post-splenectomy, not Heinz bodies.

92   a) True   b) True   c) True   d) False   e) True

Other features in congenital rubella are growth retardation, acute encephalitis, hepatitis, mental retardation, retinopathy, glaucoma and congenital heart diseases. Cerebral calcifications occur in congenital toxoplasmosis and cytomegalovirus infections.

93   a) True   b) False   c) False   d) True   e) False

Hyperacusis is seen in Tay–Sach's disease. Repeated self-mutilation is characteristic of Lesch–Nyhan syndrome. Corneal opacity is a feature in Hurler's syndrome.

94   **a) True**   **b) True**   **c) True**   **d) False**   **e) False**

Haemophilia A (factor VIII deficiency) and B (factor IX deficiency) are X-linked recessive, but haemophilia C (factor XI deficiency) is autosomal recessive. Hypochondroplasia, like achondroplasia, is autosomal dominant with sporadic cases.

95   **a) True**   **b) False**   **c) True**   **d) True**   **e) True**

The appetite can be increased as well as decreased in depression. Difficulty in falling asleep is characteristic of anxiety while early morning wakening is characteristic of depression. The weight can be increased or decreased. Feelings of worthlessness and hopelessness are the two cardinal signs of depression.

96   **a) True**   **b) False**   **c) False**   **d) False**   **e) False**

The inspiratory whoop can be absent, especially in infants. Death in pertussis is mostly due to secondary bacterial infections. The yield of isolating *Bordetella pertussis* is higher in the catarrhal phase, when the patient may not attend for advice, and when the doctor does not suspect pertussis.

97   **a) True**   **b) False**   **c) False**   **d) False**   **e) True**

An inherited failure of fusion of images, and visual impairments such as cataracts and refractive errors, give a non-paralytic concomitant squint. Raised intracranial pressure leads to sixth cranial nerve palsy (as a false localizing sign) and causes a paralytic inconcomitant squint.

98   **a) True**   **b) False**   **c) True**   **d) False**   **e) True**

99   **a) True**   **b) False**   **c) False**   **d) True**   **e) True**

Inorganic failure to thrive and radar gaze (the eyes of the child steadily following others with little head movement) are typical signs of emotional abuse and neglect. Deprivation hands and feet are cold and swollen.

100   **a) False**   **b) False**   **c) False**   **d) True**   **e) True**

The stature is initially tall for congenital adrenal hyperplasia. Because of early fusion of growth plates, the final adult height may be decreased.

101   **a) False**   **b) True**   **c) True**   **d) False**   **e) False**

102   **a) True**   **b) False**   **c) False**   **d) True**   **e) False**

Spontaneous bleeding is likely only if factor VIII is less than 5 units/dl. Paracetamol is usually adequate for joint pains. APTT is increased as the intrinsic pathway is affected.

103   a) True   b) False   c) False   d) True   e) False

Sturge–Weber syndrome is a sporadic condition. Ataxia-telangiectasia is autosomal recessive. Both neurofibromatosis-1 (chromosome 17) and neurofibromatosis-2 (chromosome 22) are autosomal dominant. They are best regarded as separate diseases. There are many types of ectodermal dysplasia. The commonest type diagnosed (it is likely that most milder types are undiagnosed) is anhidrotic ED, which is X-linked recessive.

104   a) True   b) False   c) True   d) True   e) True

Most vaccines can be given by the intramuscular or deep subcutaneous routes. BCG can only be given intradermally.

105   a) True   b) False   c) True   d) True   e) True

Other useful investigations are antigliadin antibodies, renal function tests and chromosomal analysis. X-rays of the legs and feet are useful for children below 18 months of age for bone age estimation.

106   a) True   b) False   c) False   d) True   e) False

The pulse is collapsing and the apical impulse is prominent in patent ductus arteriosus.

107   a) True   b) False   c) False   d) True   e) True

The surveillance of children in care is the responsibility of the social worker. The practice nurse is usually responsible for procedures such as ear syringing.

108   a) False   b) True   c) False   d) True   e) False

Only 1 point is given for a pulse less than 100/min. A score of 2 at 10 minutes indicates cerebral injury or likely death. The lowest possible score is zero.

109   a) True   b) True   c) False   d) True   e) False

In practice, the Emergency Protection Order is usually applied by the social worker or NSPCC staff. A contact order requires that person living with the child to allow contact with another named person. A supervision order is enforceable for 1 year initially.

110   a) True   b) False   c) True   d) False   e) True

111   a) True   b) False   c) True   d) True   e) True

Wound management is the responsibility of the district nurse or the practice nurse.

112   a) False   b) False   c) True   d) False   e) False

113   a) True   b) False   c) True   d) True   e) True

Methylphenidate has been used in the treatment of hyperactivity disorder.

114	a) False	b) True	c) False	d) True	e) True

115	a) True	b) False	c) False	d) False	e) True

High fever and bloody diarrhoea suggest that a bacterial cause is more likely.

116	a) False	b) True	c) False	d) False	e) True

Note that there are many false indications for circumcision, operation for tongue tie, and tonsillectomy and adenoidectomy.

117	a) True	b) True	c) True	d) True	e) True

118	a) True	b) True	c) True	d) False	e) False

Hand reaching beyond the tip of shoulder is the scarf sign. Incomplete wrist flexion is the window sign. Both are characteristic for a preterm baby. Legs not being flat on the couch when lying supine and high pelvis when lying prone are findings in a term baby. Note that the presence of paralytic and non-paralytic hypotonia has to be taken into account in the interpretation of such findings.

119	a) True	b) False	c) False	d) False	e) True

The reflex arc of the knee jerk passes through L3 L4, the ankle jerk S1 S2 and the cremasteric reflex L1 L2.

120	a) False	b) False	c) True	d) False	e) False

The bleeding time is normal or increased in von Willebrand's disease as there is impaired platelet aggregation. In deficiencies of factors VIII, IX, X and XI, the vessels and platelets are not involved. Thus the bleeding time is normal.

121 The following features are characteristic of pauciarticular JCA:

a) Hepatosplenomegaly
b) Positive anti-nuclear antibody
c) Positive rheumatoid factor
d) Positive HLA B27
e) Uveitis

122 Contraindications to the pertussis vaccine are:

a) High fever
b) Infantile spasm
c) Severe generalized reaction to a previous dose
d) History of Reye's syndrome
e) Epilepsy

123 A 15-year-old boy has frequency and dysuria for 2 days. Mid-stream urine shows numerous white cells with no gram-negative intracellular diplococci. Culture yielded insignificant growth. Possible causes are:

a) *Chlamydia trachomatis*
b) *Ureaplasma urealyticum*
c) *Trichomonas vaginalis*
d) Herpes simplex type 1
e) Herpes simplex type 2

124 Common causes of seizures after early infancy are:

a) Meningitis
b) Febrile convulsion
c) Reye's syndrome
d) Epilepsy
e) Cerebral tumour

125 The following diseases can now be diagnosed prenatally:

a) Sickle cell disease
b) Maple syrup urine disease
c) Retinoblastoma
d) Hypophosphaturia
e) Von Willebrand's disease

126 The variables in the Jarman index include:

a) Chronic illness
b) People on income support
c) Unemployed people
d) Overcrowded households
e) Ethnic minorities

127 An 8-year-old boy presents with slow, progressive weakness of the muscles of the ankle and feet with pes cavus. On examination the thighs look like inverted champagne bottles. Knee and ankle jerks are absent. No sensory loss is demonstrated. The diagnosis is:

a) Myasthenia gravis
b) Cerebral palsy
c) Charcot–Marie–Tooth disease
d) Duchenne muscular dystrophy
e) Werding–Hoffman disease

128 The following associations are true:

a) Phenobarbital and grand mal
b) Carbamazepam and temporal lobe epilepsy
c) Phenytoin and focal epilepsy
d) Valproate and focal epilepsy
e) Ethosuximide and petit mal

129 In head injuries, a child should be admitted for close observation in the following circumstances:

a) Projectile vomiting
b) Loss of consciousness
c) Immediate crying after injury
d) Fall on to a hard surface for a 7-year-old child
e) Fall from a height of 30 cm to the ground

130 Features of hypoplastic left heart include:

a) Prominent apex impulse
b) Weak pulses
c) Hepatomegaly
d) Gallop rhythm
e) Oligaemic lung fields

131 Examples of X-linked dominant conditions include:

a) Vitamin D resistant rickets
b) Pseudohypoparathyroidism
c) Lesch–Nyhan syndrome
d) Rett syndrome
e) Wiscott–Aldrich syndrome

132 For the diet of pre-school children:

a) Decreased total fat intake is recommended
b) Decreased sugar intake is recommended
c) Fresh fruit and raw vegetables are recommended as good snacks
d) The avoidance of excessive salt intake is recommended
e) Full fat milk is recommended

133 **Complications of tonsillitis include:**

a) Peritonsillar abscess
b) Retropharyngeal abscess
c) Glomerulonephritis
d) Rheumatic fever
e) Otitis media

134 **A 10-day-old female infant presents with repeated vomiting. Examination reveals clitoromegaly. Her serum sodium is 124 mmol/l and potassium 6.7 mmol/l. The most likely diagnosis is:**

a) Partial deficiency of 21-hydroxylase
b) Complete deficiency of 21-hydroxylase
c) Deficiency of 11-hydroxylase
d) Deficiency of 17 alpha-hydroxylase
e) Deficiency of 20 desmolase

135 **Features suggesting a chronic nature of childhood asthma are:**

a) Pectus carinatum
b) Use of accessory muscles
c) Pulsus paradoxicus
d) Harrison's sulci
e) Inspiratory breath sound

136 **In attico-antral disease:**

a) The perforation is in the pars flaccida
b) The discharge is scanty but offensive
c) Nasal polyps are associated
d) The organisms are usually Gram-positive
e) Surgical exploration of the mastoid is often indicated

137 **Drugs to be avoided in children with G6PD deficiency are:**

a) Phenacetin
b) Paracetamol
c) Sulphapyridine
d) Cefuroxime
e) Nitrofurantoin

138 **Causes of paralytic hypotonia are:**

a) Failure to thrive
b) Rickets
c) Hypercalcaemia
d) Down's syndrome
e) Hypothyroidism

139 Causes of hypernatraemia include:

a) Inappropriate antidiuretic hormone secretion
b) Diabetes insipidus
c) Nephrotic syndrome
d) Hyperaldosteronism
e) Renal tubular acidosis

140 Köebner phenomenon is demonstrated in:

a) Lichen simplex
b) Discoid eczema
c) Psoriasis
d) Secondary syphilis
e) Pityriasis alba

141 Common causes of seizures in the neonatal period include:

a) Intracranial haemorrhage
b) Electrolyte disturbances
c) Infections
d) Drug withdrawal
e) Febrile convulsion

142 Common causes of arthralgia include:

a) Rickets
b) Transient synovitis
c) Leukaemia
d) Trauma
e) Haemophilia

143 The following features suggest drug taking in adolescents:

a) Disappearance of money in the house
b) Sudden unexplained episodes of irritability
c) Increased appetite
d) Loss of interest in former hobbies and school work
e) slurred speech with blurring of vision

144 A 3-year-old boy has just had a documented urinary tract infection. Indications for a micturating cystourethrogram include:

a) Abnormal ultrasound results
b) Pyelonephritis
c) Family history of reflux
d) Recurrent infections
e) Abnormal DMSA scan result

145 An 11-year-old boy presents with diffuse bone pain, polyuria and poly-dipsia. Examination reveals exophthalmos, and extensive seborrhoeic dermatitis with evidence of mastoiditis. The most likely diagnosis is:

a) Lymphoma
b) Histiocytosis X
c) Hyperparathyroidism
d) Leukaemia
e) Medulloblastoma

146 Secondary reflexes include:

a) Downward parachute reflex
b) Neck righting reflex
c) Stepping reflex
d) Forward parachute reflex
e) Galant reflex

147 Complications of the BCG vaccination include:

a) Keloid formation
b) Anaphylaxis
c) Disseminated infection
d) Local abscess
e) Thrombocytopenia

148 Causes of unconjugated neonatal hyperbilirubinaemia include:

a) Choledochal cyst
b) Crigler–Najjar syndrome
c) Elliptocytosis
d) Breast milk jaundice
e) Hypothyroidism

149 In Reye's syndrome:

a) The basic pathology is fatty degeneration of the liver with encephalopathy
b) Chicken pox and influenza have been implicated as precipitating factors
c) Hypoglycaemia is usual
d) Raised liver transaminases are usual
e) Jaundice is usual

150 A child refuses to retire to bed:

a) He should be allowed to sleep in his parents' bed
b) The light of his bedroom must be turned off
c) The door of his bedroom can be left open to make him feel safe
d) Reasonable sleep routine is helpful
e) If he cries in bed, he should be ignored

151 **In pyloric stenosis:**

a) Presentation is typical in the second week of life
b) First-born males are more commonly affected
c) Feeding refusal is common
d) Weight loss and dehydration are characteristic
e) A family history is present in 50% of cases

152 **A neonate develops jaundice on day 3. The colour of the stool and urine is normal. He continues to breastfeed satisfactorily. The following measures should be employed:**

a) Continue the breastfeeding
b) Stop the breastfeeding
c) Check the bilirubin level
d) Start phototherapy
e) Reassure the parents

153 **Features in the background of a male homosexual might include:**

a) Prolonged absence of the father in the first 5 years
b) Hostility to the mother
c) The father sleeping with him
d) Parental favouritism towards the boy's brother
e) Undue attachment to the father

154 **For the social classes:**

a) Social class 1 includes the major professionals and higher administrative staff
b) Social class 2 involves the lesser professionals, administrative and managerial staff
c) Social class 3 includes the clerical and skilled workers
d) Social class 4 includes the skilled manual workers
e) Social class 5 includes the semi-skilled workers

155 **Reliable signs of heart failure in a child include:**

a) Tachycardia
b) Collapse and shock
c) Basal crepitations
d) Longer time needed for feeding
e) Raised jugular venous pulse

156 **The following diseases can now be diagnosed antenatally:**

a) Hypercholesterolaemia
b) Polycystic kidney disease
c) Cystinosis
d) Gaucher's disease
e) Beta thalassaemia

157 **In urine collection:**

a) Results are difficult to interpret for bag urine samples
b) A suprapubic tap is a highly dangerous procedure
c) An ultrasound machine must be available for a suprapubic tap
d) A positive culture greater than 10^5 organisms/ml in a midstream urine is diagnostic of urinary tract infection
e) Routine microurinalysis is not recommended in pre-school medical examinations

158 **Recommendations to prevent iron deficiency include:**

a) Tea as a diet supplement
b) Not giving cows' milk to infants under 1 year
c) Routine screening for all children
d) Iron supplements for all infants
e) Weaning to mixed feeding after 8 months of age

159 **A 1-year-old child can:**

a) Unzip fasteners
b) Climb on hands and feet
c) Walk backwards in imitation
d) Build a tower of 3 bricks
e) Shuffle on buttocks and hands

160 **The following are compatible with a diagnosis of nephrotic syndrome:**

a) Proteinuria more than 20 mg/h/m^2
b) Plasma albumin 20 g/l
c) Plasma albumin 18 g/l
d) Hypercholesterolaemia
e) Peripheral oedema

161 **Features which differentiate acute epiglottitis from croup are:**

a) Hoarse voice
b) Barking cough
c) Aged 3 or above
d) Drooling of saliva
e) Normal chest X-ray

162 **In endocardial fibroelastosis:**

a) Pulses are characteristically weak
b) Central cyanosis is virtually always present
c) A fibrotic small heart is characteristic
d) Hepatomegaly is unusual
e) Spontaneous regression may occur

163 Measures to prevent burns at home include:

a) Dressing the child in a suitable nightdress
b) Placing mirrors near the fire
c) Not allowing a child to play with matches
d) Not leaving an electric iron plugged in
e) Not letting the child hold a firework

164 The following features support a diagnosis of school refusal rather than truancy:

a) Poor academic record
b) Stable family background
c) Being the only child in the family
d) Of a younger age
e) History of fire setting

165 Adverse factors in single-parent families include:

a) Detached relationships
b) Financial constraints
c) Lack of modelling of male/female relationships
d) Less emotional support for the parent
e) Social adversity

166 A 2-year-old girl, staying in a nursery, was admitted and diagnosed to have meningitis due to *Haemophilus influenzae* type b. She had not received the Hib vaccination before.

a) Her brother, aged 1, should receive 1 dose of the Hib vaccine even if he has received 3 doses at 2, 3 and 4 months
b) The index case should receive 3 doses of Hib vaccine later
c) Other children in the nursery, aged 4 or below, should be given rifampicin even if they are fully immunized
d) If 1 further case of invasive Hib disease occurs in the nursery 30 days later, all the staff and children in the nursery should be given rifampicin
e) A child in the nursery is asplenic. This is not a contraindication for Hib vaccination

167 Causes of in-toeing are:

a) Metatarsus varus
b) Tibial torsion
c) Femoral anteversion
d) Femoral retroversion
e) Knock knee

168 Advantages of normal schools in contrast to special schools include:

a) Normal role models
b) Local contacts for parents
c) Nearer to the homes of the children
d) Normal expectation
e) Large classes

169 Risk factors for child abuse include:

a) Presence of step-parent
b) History of drug addiction
c) History of family violence
d) A physically handicapped infant
e) Infant separated from mother for less than 24 hours

170 Influenza:

a) Is caused by rhinovirus
b) Is transmitted by droplet spread
c) Has an incubation period of 7 to 14 days
d) Can be complicated by myocarditis and encephalomyelitis
e) Can be prevented by Hib vaccination

171 For good dental health:

a) Sugary foods should be avoided
b) Fluoride from the water supply, supplementary drops or toothpaste are helpful
c) A concentration of 1 ppm fluoride in drinking water is adequate
d) Brushing and washing of teeth should start at the age of 2
e) Whether the child needs milk late at night should be considered in the history

172 A 1-year-old child develops anaphylaxis 4 hours after MMR vaccination. The following medications might be useful:

a) Adrenaline 1/1000 0.5 ml intramuscularly
b) Adrenaline 1/1000 0.1 ml subcutaneously
c) Chlopheniramine 2.5 mg slow intravenously
d) Hydrocortisone 100 mg slow intravenously
e) Hydrocortisone 500 mg slow intravenously

173 In diabetes in children:

a) A high fat, low sugar, high fibre diet is recommended
b) Normal amounts of carbohydrates are recommended
c) Traditional eating patterns in ethnic groups should be respected
d) 'Amber' in the traffic light system means foods high in refined carbohydrates
e) 'Green' in the traffic light system means foods free of carbohydrates

174 **The following statements are true:**

a) Accidents are the commonest cause of death in children older than 1 year
b) Fire is the commonest cause of mortality in accidents
c) Most fatal road accidents occur in the afternoon
d) Boys are more likely than girls to be the victims of fatal road accidents
e) Foreign body ingestion/inhalation is the commonest accident in the home

175 **In myocarditis:**

a) Coxsackie B virus is a common cause
b) Occurrence in infancy is rare
c) Muffled heart sounds are characteristic
d) ECG shows T wave inversions in V4–V6
e) Echocardiogram usually reveals no abnormality

176 **A 15-year-old girl is suspected to have Turner's syndrome. The following are compatible with the diagnosis:**

a) History of puffy hands and feet at birth
b) Absence of neck webbing
c) Chromosomal analysis showing 46XX/45XO mosaicism
d) History of menstruation
e) Not of short stature

177 **A newborn infant has central cyanosis and fits with slow and shallow breathing. A nitrogen wash-out test produces a slight rise in the PO_2. The most likely cause for the cyanosis is:**

a) Methaemoglobinaemia
b) Cerebral disorder
c) Persistent fetal circulation
d) Congenital cyanotic heart disease
e) Lung disease

178 **Haemophilia A is associated with:**

a) Pseudotumours of bone
b) Muscle haematomas
c) Degeneration of joints
d) Muscle wasting
e) Haemarthrosis

179 **The following are compatible with a diagnosis of pertussis:**

a) A local epidemic
b) Previous history of immunization
c) Overinflation in the chest X-ray
d) A normal chest X-ray
e) Lymphocytosis

180 **In Ebstein anomaly:**

a) Mitral regurgitation is usually present
b) Central cyanosis is characteristic
c) Wolff–Parkinson–White syndrome is associated
d) Lung plethora is usual
e) Left bundle branch block is usual

121   a) False   b) True   c) False   d) True   e) True

Hepatosplenomegaly is characteristic of Still's disease. Positive anti-nuclear antibody is characteristic of the 'younger girls' variety of pauciarticular JCA, while positive HLA B27 is characteristic of the 'older boys' variety of pauciarticular JCA. Some patients with polyarticular JCA have positive rheumatoid factor. They can be said to have 'childhood rheumatoid arthritis' or 'Juvenile rheumatoid arthritis'.

122   a) True   b) False   c) True   d) False   e) False

If the child is febrile, vaccination should be postponed. A documented or reliable history of severe local or generalized reaction to a previous dose is a true contraindication, while the others are false contraindications.

123   a) True   b) True   c) True   d) True   e) True

Chlamydia trachomatis serovars D-K is the commonest cause of non-gonococcal urethritis. Excluding Gonococcus and Chlamydia, *Ureaplasma urealyticum* is the commonest cause of non-specific urethritis, for which *Trichomonas vaginalis* and the herpes simplex viruses are also causes. Note that in genital infections, herpes type 1 can be responsible for as many as 30–35% of cases, with herpes 2 causing 65–70% of cases of herpes infections.

124   a) True   b) True   c) False   d) True   e) False

Reye's syndrome can cause seizures but the disease itself is uncommon. Cerebral tumour is rare.

125   a) True   b) True   c) True   d) True   e) True

126   a) False   b) False   c) True   d) True   e) True

The Jarman index describes eight variables which increase the workload of general practitioners. The other variables are: old people living alone, children under 5, single parents, unskilled people and people who have moved house.

127   a) False   b) False   c) True   d) False   e) False

The history and findings are suggestive of progressive peripheral neuropathy. Thus, peroneal muscular atrophy is the likely diagnosis. Note that the sensory loss is uncommon in childhood.

128   a) True   b) True   c) True   d) False   e) True

Both primidone and phenobarbital can be used for grand mal, as the former is partly metabolized to the latter. Sodium valproate is used for grand mal and absence seizures.

129   a) True   b) True   c) False   d) False   e) False

130   a) False   b) True   c) True   d) True   e) False

In hypoplastic left heart, the right ventricular impulse is prominent and a parasternal heave may be present. Heart failure is early and leads to hepatomegaly and gallop rhythm. The lung fields show venous congestion.

131   a) True   b) True   c) False   d) True   e) False

Both Lesch–Nyhan and Wiscott–Aldrich syndromes are X-linked recessive.

132   a) False   b) True   c) True   d) True   e) True

Guidelines for adults and schoolchildren should not be extended to the pre-school child. Thus a decreased total fat intake has not been recommended. Decreased sugar intake is recommended to prevent dental caries. Full fat milk should be given to the pre-school child rather than skimmed milk, although semi-skimmed milk can be slowly introduced.

133   a) True   b) True   c) True   d) True   e) True

134   a) False   b) True   c) False   d) False   e) False

Decreased 21-hydroxylase is the 'pure virilizing' form. Complete deficiency of 21-hydroxylase is the 'salt losing' form. 11-hydroxylase deficiency is the 'hypertensive' form. 17 alpha-hydroxylase deficiency leads to salt retention, not salt losing. 20-desmolase deficiency leads to salt losing. However, there is no clitoromegaly.

135   a) True   b) False   c) False   d) True   e) False

Pulsus paradoxicus is now shown to be of little use in the indication of the severity of an asthma attack. It is not related to the chronicity of the condition.

136   a) True   b) True   c) False   d) False   e) True

Aural polyps are associated with the attico-antral disease. The organisms are mainly gram-negative.

137   a) True   b) False   c) True   d) False   e) True

138   a) False   b) False   c) False   d) False   e) False

All are good examples of causes of non-paralytic hypotonia.

139   a) False   b) True   c) False   d) True   e) False

SIADH, nephrotic syndrome and renal tubular acidosis are causes of hyponatraemia.

140   a) False   b) False   c) True   d) False   e) False

In psoriasis, the lesions may appear in sites of previous trauma, i.e. the Köebner phenomenon. This phenomenon is also seen with viral warts and lichen planus. Some dermatologists, however, insist that the Köebner phenomenon should be limited to a pressure effect, not transmission of an infective agent by trauma, and thus exclude viral warts as a disease demonstrating the phenomenon.

141   a) True   b) True   c) True   d) True   e) False

Febrile convulsions occur at 6 months to 5 years only.

142   a) False   b) True   c) False   d) True   e) False

Rickets is rare in developed countries. Haemophilia is uncommon and leukaemia is rare.

143   a) True   b) True   c) False   d) True   e) True

A loss of appetite is typically associated.

144   a) True   b) True   c) True   d) True   e) True

145   a) False   b) True   c) False   d) False   e) False

Osteolytic bone lesions, diabetes insipidus, exophthalmos, mastoiditis and seborrhoeic-dermatitis-like rash all point to Hand–Schuller–Christian disease.

146   a) True   b) True   c) False   d) True   e) False

147   a) True   b) True   c) True   d) True   e) False

Thrombocytopenia is a very rare complication of rubella vaccination.

148   a) False   b) True   c) True   d) True   e) True

Choledochal cyst leads to conjugated hyperbilirubinaemia.

149   a) True   b) True   c) True   d) True   e) False

Bilirubin is usually normal in Reye's syndrome.

150   a) False   b) True   c) False   d) True   e) True

The child must not be allowed to sleep with his parents. Otherwise, he will think that sleeping alone is fearful. The bedroom light must be turned off, or he will think that darkness is unsafe. Opening the bedroom door is just inviting him to come out. Sleep routines help to prepare the child to sleep. Excessive routine, however, should be avoided. If he cries in bed, after making sure that he is safe, the crying should be ignored. The neighbours should be warned beforehand, though.

151   a) False   b) True   c) False   d) True   e) False

Pyloric stenosis usually presents at 2 to 6 weeks. The baby does not refuse feeding. He may look even hungrier than usual. A family history is present in only 15–20% of cases.

152   a) True   b) False   c) True   d) False   e) True

153   a) True   b) False   c) False   d) False   e) False

Hostility to the father, sleeping with the mother, parental favouritism towards the boy's sister and undue attachment to the mother are factors.

154   a) True   b) True   c) True   d) False   e) False

Examples for major professionals are medical practitioners and solicitors. Teachers and registered nurses are lesser professionals. Class 3 is divided into class 3N (skilled non-manual) and class 3M (skilled manual). Class 4 includes the semi-skilled occupations and class 5 the unskilled occupations and labourers. The social class of a housewife follows that of her husband.

155   a) True   b) True   c) False   d) True   e) False

156   a) True   b) True   c) True   d) True   e) True

157   a) True   b) False   c) False   d) True   e) True

Bag urine samples are contaminated to a certain extent and interpretation is difficult. The suprapubic tap is safe under experienced hands. The confirmation of a full bladder by ultrasound before tapping is desirable, but not absolutely necessary. Routine microurinalysis does not fulfil the criteria of a cost-effective screening test.

158   a) False   b) True   c) False   d) False   e) False

Iron supplements to all infants is currently not recommended in the UK. Weaning to mixed feeding should start at 4 to 6 months.

159   a) False   b) True   c) False   d) False   e) True

Most children can unzip fasteners, walk backwards in imitation and build a tower of 3 bricks at 18 months. 'Bottom-shufflers' are common and may have delayed walking. Other aspects of development are not affected.

160   a) False   b) True   c) True   d) True   e) True

The proteinuria is more than 40 mg/hr/m^2

161 a) False b) False c) True d) True e) False

A hoarse voice and a normal chest X-ray can occur in both croup and acute epiglottitis. A barking cough is characteristic of croup. There is usually no cough in acute epiglottitis. Drooling of saliva is very characteristic of acute epiglottitis.

162 a) True b) False c) False d) False e) True

There is no central cyanosis as there is no right-to-left shunt. The heart is dilated with hypertrophy.

163 a) False b) False c) True d) True e) True

The child should be dressed in pyjamas rather than a nightdress. Mirrors placed near the fire might attract the attention of a child.

164 a) False b) True c) True d) True e) False

The risk factors, characteristics, prognosis and plan associated with the management of school refusal are almost totally different from those of truancy. Poor academic record and a history of stealing or fire setting are supportive of truancy. The incidence of school phobia increases up the social classes while that of truancy increases down the social classes.

165 a) False b) True c) True d) True e) True

Relationships in single-parent families are likely to be over-involved rather than detached. Social adversity is common, leading to a chain of disadvantages.

166 a) False b) False c) False d) True e) True

The index case should receive one injection only, as should any unimmunized child aged 13 to 48 months. Rifampicin prophylaxis is not needed if only one case occurs and the children are fully immunized. However, if two or more cases occur within 120 days, all the staff and children should receive rifampicin 20 mg/kg/day for 4 days.

167 a) True b) True c) True d) False e) False

Tibial torsion can cause both in-and out-toeing. Femoral retroversion is a cause of out-toeing. Knock knee is more often associated with out-toeing.

168 a) True b) True c) True d) True e) False

169 a) True b) True c) True d) True e) False

Separation from mother for more than 24 hours is a risk factor for child abuse.

170 a) False b) True c) False d) True e) False

Influenzae A, B and C are orthomyxoviruses. The incubation period is 2 to 3 days. Influenza vaccine, not Hib vaccine, gives about 70% protection and has to be given annually to indicated cases.

171   a) True   b) True   c) True   d) False   e) True

As soon as there are teeth, the mother may 'brush' or wash them gently. If the child needs milk very late at night, the teeth must be cleaned afterwards.

172   a) False   b) True   c) True   d) False   e) False

Hydrocortisone 25 mg, slow intravenously, should be administered.

173   a) False   b) True   c) True   d) False   e) True

The recommended diet is low fat, low sugar, high fibre. Normal amounts of carbohydrates are recommended, but most should be unrefined. With the help of a dietician, traditional eating patterns should be respected as far as possible. 'Amber' in the traffic light system means carbohydrate exchanges. 'Red' means foods high in refined carbohydrates.

174   a) True   b) False   c) True   d) True   e) False

Road traffic accidents are the commonest cause of death in accidents. Falls are the commonest accident in the home.

175   a) True   b) False   c) True   d) True   e) False

The echocardiogram reveals a dilated, poorly contracting heart in myocarditis.

176   a) True   b) True   c) True   d) False   e) True

Neck webbing is not necessarily present to make the diagnosis. All have amenorrhoea. The girl may not be excessively short if she has tall parents.

177   a) False   b) True   c) False   d) False   e) False

The fits with shallow breathing point to a CNS diagnosis.

178   a) True   b) True   c) True   d) True   e) True

179   a) True   b) True   c) False   d) True   e) True

The protection from immunization is not absolute. A hyperinflated chest on a chest X-ray is suggestive of acute bronchiolitis. The chest X-ray in pertussis is usually normal, though small areas of collapse/consolidation may sometimes be seen.

180   a) False   b) True   c) True   d) False   e) False

Tricuspid regurgitation is present in Ebstein anomaly, not mitral regurgitation. The lung fields are oligaemic. Right bundle branch block is often present.

181 **Prune belly syndrome:**

a) Is associated with polyhydramnios
b) Is associated with pulmonary hypoplasia
c) Presents with central cyanosis
d) Is more prevalent in females
e) Is associated with undescended testes

182 **In total anomalous pulmonary venous drainage:**

a) Central cyanosis is incompatible with the diagnosis
b) Symptoms usually develop in the newborn period
c) A venous hum is present in almost every case
d) Cardiomegaly is often present
e) ECG is often normal

183 **For weaning:**

a) Weaning must be started at 3 to 4 months
b) Early weaning might predispose the infant to infection and sensitization
c) Late weaning might lead to inadequate nutrition
d) New foods should be introduced one at a time
e) The amount given should initially be very small

184 **A $1\frac{1}{2}$-year-old child presents with unilateral, greenish nasal discharge which is bloodstained and offensive:**

a) X-ray of the paranasal sinuses is indicated
b) Steroid nasal spray is indicated
c) A trial of oral antihistamine is needed
d) Serum IgE level is helpful
e) General anaesthesia might be needed

185 **Innocent murmurs:**

a) Are constant
b) Only occur in the systolic phase
c) Usually become louder when the child stands up
d) Are associated with normal chest X-ray and ECG
e) Are exacerbated by fever

186 **Conditions associated with oligohydramnios include:**

a) Infantile polycystic kidney
b) Congenital heart disease
c) Intrauterine growth retardation
d) High intestinal obstruction
e) Posterior urethral valves

187 **According to the DHSS (1984) report:**

a) No more than 35% of food energy should come from fat
b) No more than 25% of food energy should come from saturated fats
c) Complex carbohydrates are preferred to simple carbohydrates
d) Excessive salt intake should be avoided
e) The report applies to children over 2 years and adults

188 **Drugs which can be safely taken by a child with G6PD deficiency include:**

a) Primaquine
b) Chloramphenicol
c) Probenecid
d) Nalidixic acid
e) Chloroquine

189 **Characteristic features in the coarctation of the aorta include:**

a) Variable systolic murmur over the precordium
b) Hypertension in the arms
c) An association with Noonan's syndrome
d) The narrowing being proximal to the origin of the left subclavian artery
e) X-ray showing rib notching in infants

190 **In plaque psoriasis:**

a) Topical steroids are safe and effective
b) Soft paraffin is useful
c) Coal tar is useful
d) Most will be exacerbated by sunlight
e) Dithranol is poorly tolerated in children

191 **The following are associated with infantile spasms:**

a) Tuberous sclerosis
b) Neonatal hypoxia
c) Congenital toxoplasma infection
d) Neurofibromatosis-1
e) Phenylketonuria

192 **In the CSF in a 3-year-old child:**

a) Partially treated bacterial meningitis usually gives a clear appearance
b) Polymorphs may account for 50% of the white cell count in early viral meningitis
c) Polymerase chain reaction may assist the diagnosis of tuberculous meningitis
d) The glucose level is often very low in tuberculous meningitis
e) A protein level of 3.7 g/l suggests bacterial or tuberculous meningitis

193 **To promote breastfeeding, one should:**

a) Start breastfeeding on day 3 so as to give the mother adequate rest
b) Give supplementary feeds to avoid underfeeding
c) Encourage feeding at set times
d) Insist on breastfeeding even if the mother objects
e) Not give samples of infant formula to mothers

194 **Causes of acute prerenal failure include:**

a) Gentamicin
b) Sulphonamides
c) Haemolytic uraemic syndrome
d) Reye's syndrome
e) Renal vein thrombosis

195 **The following medications can be safely taken while breastfeeding:**

a) Cimetidine
b) Co-trimoxazole
c) Propanolol
d) Chlormethiazole
e) Codeine

196 **The ECG of a 4-month-old infant shows a regular heart rate of 240/min with normal QRS complexes and no P waves:**

a) Diving reflex can be attempted
b) Adenosine can be given at 1 mg/kg IV bolus
c) Verapamil should be used only if adenosine fails to return the heart to sinus rhythm
d) Verapamil should be used only if propanolol is also being administered
e) DC cardioversion may be needed

197 **The following associations are true:**

a) Thromboembolism and Marfan's syndrome
b) Normal intelligence and Marfan's syndrome
c) Osteoporosis and Marfan's syndrome
d) Downward lens subluxation and homocystinuria
e) Autosomal recessiveness and homocystinuria

198 **In the management of paraquat poisoning:**

a) Emesis may be induced
b) Gastric lavage may be indicated
c) Purgation may be indicated
d) Suspension of Fuller's earth BPC is helpful
e) Activated charcoal is helpful

199 **Opportunities for primary prevention in a child health promotion service include:**

a) Increase uptake of immunization
b) Prevention of SIDS
c) Prevention of child abuse
d) Screening for iron deficiency anaemia
e) Promotion of dental health

200 **A newborn infant has breathing difficulty with central cyanosis. A nitrogen washout test raised the PO_2 to 15 kPa. Possible diagnoses include:**

a) Fallot's tetralogy
b) Ventricular septal defect
c) Pneumonia
d) Tricuspid atresia
e) Hyaline membrane disease

201 **The Moro reflex:**

a) Is present at birth
b) Is a secondary reflex
c) Disappears around 5 months
d) Can be asymmetric in brachial plexus injury
e) If persisting beyond 3 months is suggestive of a neuromuscular disorder

202 **The following are relevant in megaloblastic anaemia:**

a) History of epilepsy
b) History of intestinal resection
c) History of hypothyroidism
d) History of coeliac disease
e) Teenage pregnancy

203 **Resuscitation of a neonate with coarctation of the aorta might require the use of:**

a) Frusemide
b) Bicarbonate
c) Indomethacin
d) Dopamine
e) Prostaglandin E

204 An 18-month-old boy has had grossly delayed motor development since birth. He is hypotonic with intentional tremor. A prominent occiput is noted. The likely diagnosis is:

a) Cerebellar abscess
b) Ataxia telangiectasia
c) Lead poisoning
d) Cerebellar tumour
e) Dandy–Walker syndrome

205 Reliable signs of heart failure in a child include:

a) Sweating on feeding
b) Ankle oedema
c) Breathlessness on feeding and exertion
d) Tachypnoea
e) Hepatomegaly

206 The following conditions are associated with a monophonic wheeze:

a) Asthma
b) Inhaled foreign body
c) Vascular ring
d) Cystic fibrosis
e) Aspiration pneumonia

207 A child has a sudden onset of petechiae on the extensor surface of the buttocks and lower limbs. There is associated abdominal pain. The following are expected findings:

a) Migratory polyarthralgia
b) Thrombocytopenia
c) Permanent damage to the joints
d) Haematuria
e) Gastrointestinal bleeding

208 The Personal Child Health Record should include:

a) Phenylketonuria and hypothyroidism entries
b) Checklist for injury prevention
c) Information about screening
d) Nine-centile growth charts
e) Developmental yes/no checklists

209 **Causes of regular (smooth) hepatomegaly include:**

a) Choledochal cyst
b) Neuroblastoma
c) Hydatid cyst
d) Nephroblastoma
e) Cardiac failure

210 **In cyanotic congenital heart diseases:**

a) Transposition of great arteries leads to increased pulmonary blood flow
b) Pulmonary blood flow is increased in tricuspid atresia
c) Pulmonary blood flow is decreased in Ebstein anomaly
d) Pulmonary blood flow is increased in hypoplastic left heart
e) Pulmonary blood flow is increased in truncus arteriosus

211 **For an X-linked recessive condition:**

a) All the sons of an affected male are affected
b) All the sons of an affected female are affected
c) Female carriers are relatively or completely normal
d) About half of the offspring of an affected male and a female carrier will manifest the condition
e) The Lyon's hypothesis helps to explain the variable penetration in some cases

212 **Differential diagnoses of asthma for a 3-year-old child include:**

a) Postnasal drip
b) Laryngotracheobronchitis
c) Tuberculosis
d) Cystic fibrosis
e) Angioneurotic oedema

213 **Causes of delayed closure of the anterior fontanelle include:**

a) Patau's syndrome
b) Hypothyroidism
c) Hydrocephalus
d) Congenital rubella
e) Rickets

214 **Eczema herpeticum:**

a) All cases are due to the human herpes virus, type 1 infection
b) Atopic eczema is the most important predisposing factor
c) Lymphadenopathy is usually present
d) It affects only one side of the body
e) Acyclovir is indicated

215 A $1\frac{1}{4}$-year-old child has chronic diarrhoea with abdominal distention. He is irritable on being examined. His height is on the 10th percentile and his weight just below the 3rd percentile. The most likely diagnosis is:

a) Coeliac disease
b) Crohn's disease
c) Ulcerative colitis
d) Cows' milk protein intolerance
e) Acrodermatitis enteropathica

216 According to the 1981 Education Act:

a) A child has 'special educational needs' if he has a learning difficulty which calls for 'special educational provision'
b) A 'Statement of Special Needs' is to be drafted
c) Children with special educational needs are to be educated in special schools with facilities to meet their needs
d) Corporal punishment in schools should be banned
e) A National Curriculum is to be introduced

217 Regarding hepatitis A:

a) It is a sexually transmissible disease
b) For children travelling to endemic areas, a single 360 ELISA units of hepatitis A vaccine should be given
c) A second injection 6 to 12 months later gives a persistent immunity up to 10 years
d) Specific immunoglobulin is available for contact cases
e) Immunization should be offered to homosexual adolescents

218 African children are more likely to have:

a) Keloids
b) Premature thelarche
c) Umbilical hernia
d) Cystic fibrosis
e) Premature pubarche

219 The external criteria of the Dubowitz score for gestational age include:

a) Nipple formation
b) Ear form and firmness
c) Skin colour and opacity
d) Protruding tongue
e) Plantar creases

220 Contraindications to live vaccines include:

a) Those on chemotherapy or radiotherapy
b) Pregnancy
c) On prophylactic, inhaled steroids
d) Immunoglobulin given 4 weeks earlier
e) Another live vaccine administered 4 weeks earlier

221 To measure height accurately:

a) A microtoise can be used
b) The outer canthus of the child's eyes should be on the same horizontal plane as the external auditory meatus
c) The examiner should exert gentle upward pressure on the child's chin
d) The child should be looking at the examiner rather than looking down
e) The standard deviation of the measurement should be no more than 1 cm

222 A 7-year-old boy was given 3 injections of hepatitis B vaccine because of close family contact. His HBsAb, 2 months after the last injection, is 185 miu/ml.

a) His HBsAg should be checked
b) His HBeAg and HBeAb should be checked
c) He is now immune to hepatitis B. The immunity is likely to be lifelong
d) A booster dose should now be given
e) A booster dose should be given 5 years later

223 A 5-year-old boy has progressive weakness and anaemia over 4 weeks. Smooth hepatosplenomegaly is present. Blood picture shows immature white cells. The diagnosis is:

a) Aplastic anaemia
b) Infectious mononucleosis
c) Acute leukaemia
d) Osteoporosis
e) HIV infection

224 An 18-month-old child can:

a) Build towers of 6 to 8 bricks
b) Turn door knobs
c) Climb stairs unaided, holding the rail
d) Walk upstairs, two feet per step
e) Turn pages one at a time

225 **A 2-year-old child can:**

a) Wash and dry hands by himself
b) Ride a tricycle
c) Turn pages one at a time
d) Unbutton large buttons
e) Walk on tiptoe when demonstrated

226 **Normal fine motor development is as follows:**

a) 4 months: hand–hand transfer
b) 6 months: palmar grasp of cube
c) 8 months: pincer grasp of small objects
d) 13 months: tower of 2 cubes
e) 18 months: feed himself with a cup

227 **The Court Report (1976) recommended that:**

a) Child health services in the community be provided by general practitioners
b) At least one Consultant Community Paediatrician per district be appointed
c) The District Handicap Team be set up
d) Sex education be made compulsory in secondary schools
e) School clinics be set up

228 **The following can cause a false negative tuberculin test:**

a) Sarcoidosis
b) MMR vaccination
c) Systemic steroids
d) Hodgkin's disease
e) HIV infection

229 **In the step-care plan of management for childhood asthma:**

a) Step 1 is the regular use of inhaled bronchodilators
b) Step 2 is the regular use of anti-inflammatory agents (e.g. cromoglycate)
c) Step 3 is the occasional use of low dose, inhaled steroids
d) Step 4 is the regular use of high dose, systemic steroids
e) Step 5 is the use of xanthines, anticholinergic agents or systemic steroids

230 **Causes of conductive hearing loss include:**

a) Neonatal jaundice
b) Treacher Collins syndrome
c) Pendred syndrome
d) Foreign body
e) Birth asphyxia

231 In the immunization schedule:

a) 2 doses of MMR are given
b) Booster Td and polio are given at 13 to 18 years
c) 4 doses of Hib are given
d) BCG is given routinely between 10 to 14 years
e) Hepatitis B is given routinely at 2, 3 and 4 months

232 Abnormal platelet functions are related to:

a) Uraemia
b) Cardiopulmonary bypass surgery
c) Aspirin
d) Dysproteinaemia
e) Bernard-Soulier disease

233 A 6-year-old boy has had nocturnal enuresis for 2 months. He has been continent since he was 2 years old:

a) A star-chart should be given as behavioural therapy
b) An electric buzzer should be given
c) DDAVP should be tried
d) Secondary causes must be ruled out first
e) He should be referred to a psychiatrist

234 The following associations are correct:

a) Chicken pox and ataxia
b) Mumps and arthralgia
c) Scarlet fever and nephritis
d) Roseola infantum and thrombocytopenia
e) Rubella and pneumonia

235 A 3-year-old child can:

a) Count up to 10
b) Copy a square
c) Unbutton large buttons
d) Button up large buttons
e) Jump off one step with two feet together

236 The following features suggest that an asthma attack is severe:

a) Peak flow rate less than 50% of the predicted or best value
b) Pulse less than 140 beats/min
c) Too breathless to talk
d) Respiration less than 50 breaths/min
e) Too breathless to feed

237 In the management of chronic childhood asthma with the step-care management plan:

a) A peak flow meter should be prescribed where possible
b) Treatment should start at step 1 and then gradually be stepped up
c) Treatment should start at step 5 and then gradually be stepped down
d) Systemic steroids can be given only at step 5
e) Regular review is needed

238 Exogenous eczema includes:

a) Atopic eczema
b) Seborrhoeic dermatitis
c) Irritant contact dermatitis
d) Pompholyx
e) Photocontact dermatitis

239 Characteristic findings in a full term baby are:

a) Full knee extension with hips fully flexed
b) Momentary neck extension when held sitting
c) Chin reaches beyond tip of shoulder
d) Hips abducted and legs flat on couch when lying supine
e) Full ankle dorsiflexion

240 The following incubation periods are true:

a) Measles: 14 to 21 days
b) Glandular fever: 2 to 4 days
c) Rubella: 14 to 21 days
d) Mumps: 10 to 14 days
e) Roseola infantum: 5 to 15 days

181 **a) False** **b) True** **c) False** **d) False** **e) True**

Prune belly syndrome is associated with oligohydramnios. There is no central cyanosis. Males are much more commonly affected.

182 **a) False** **b) True** **c) False** **d) False** **e) True**

A venous hum is one of the innocent murmurs. The heart is usually small in total anomalous pulmonary venous drainage. Central cyanosis is present in TAPVD when there is obstruction, most commonly with the infracardiac type.

183 **a) False** **b) True** **c) True** **d) True** **e) True**

Weaning, (the introduction of any food other than milk) can be started at 4 to 6 months.

184 **a) False** **b) False** **c) False** **d) False** **e) True**

The history is very suggestive of a foreign body. If it cannot be easily removed, removal under general anaesthesia may be needed.

185 **a) False** **b) False** **c) False** **d) True** **e) True**

Innocent murmurs typically change with posture and exercise. A venous hum usually extends into the diastolic phase. The innocent systolic vibratory murmur becomes louder when the child lies down and softer when he stands up.

186 **a) True** **b) False** **c) True** **d) False** **e) True**

Congenital heart diseases are not related to oligohydramnios. High intestinal obstruction is associated with polyhydramnios.

187 **a) True** **b) False** **c) True** **d) True** **e) False**

No more than 15% of food energy should come from saturated fats. Children under 5 years of age are explicitly excluded in the report.

188 **a) False** **b) False** **c) False** **d) False** **e) False**

189 **a) True** **b) True** **c) False** **d) False** **e) False**

Coarctation of the aorta is associated with Turner's syndrome. Noonan's syndrome is associated with pulmonary stenosis. The stenosis is usually distal to the origin of the left subclavian artery. Rib notching is seen in older children only.

190 **a) False** **b) True** **c) True** **d) False** **e) False**

Topical steroids are loved by many patients with plaque psoriasis as they give rapid relief, are not messy, do not irritate and do not stain wallpapers. However, their use should be discouraged as they rapidly lead to tachyphylaxis, rebound and dependence. Tar baths are useful. Dithranol is usually well tolerated in children. 90% of all cases (children and adults) will improve with sunlight, while 10% will be exacerbated by sunlight.

| 191 | a) True | b) True | c) True | d) False | e) True |

| 192 | a) True | b) True | c) True | d) True | e) True |

| 193 | a) False | b) False | c) False | d) False | e) True |

One should encourage breastfeeding very soon after delivery. Supplementary feeds should not be given easily. Such should be given only after proper test feeding to establish a diagnosis of inadequate feeding. Feeding on demand is encouraged. Only advice but not coercion should be given to promote breastfeeding. The will of the mother should always be respected. The mother should not be given any unsolicited formula milk samples.

| 194 | a) False | b) False | c) False | d) True | e) True |

Gentamicin and the haemolytic uraemic syndrome cause intrarenal failure. Sulphonamides can cause postrenal failure.

| 195 | a) True | b) False | c) False | d) True | e) True |

| 196 | a) True | b) False | c) False | d) False | e) True |

Adenosine can be given at 0.05 mg/kg increasing to a maximum dose of 0.3 mg/kg. Verapamil is not given to infants less than 1 year of age. As a calcium channel antagonist, it is contraindicated to be used concomitantly with beta-blockers.

| 197 | a) False | b) True | c) False | d) True | e) True |

Thromboembolism and osteoporosis are features of homocystinuria.

| 198 | a) True | b) True | c) True | d) True | e) True |

| 199 | a) True | b) True | c) True | d) False | e) True |

Screening for iron deficiency anaemia is a secondary preventive activity.

| 200 | a) False | b) False | c) True | d) False | e) True |

| 201 | a) True | b) False | c) True | d) True | e) False |

The Moro reflex is a primary reflex.

| 202 | a) True | b) True | c) False | d) True | e) False |

Children with a history of epilepsy may be taking anticonvulsants. Intestinal resection might lead to B12 deficiency. Hypothyroidism leads to macrocytosis with no megaloblastosis. Coeliac disease leads to combined B12 and folate deficiency. Pregnancy is associated with macrocytosis but not megaloblastosis.

67

203   a) True   b) True   c) False   d) True   e) True

Indomethacin will close the ductus arteriosus, further worsening the condition. Prostaglandin E opens the ductus arteriosus.

204   a) False   b) False   c) False   d) False   e) True

The history suggests a congenital cerebellar lesion. A prominent occiput may be present in Dandy–Walker syndrome.

205   a) True   b) False   c) True   d) True   e) True

206   a) False   b) True   c) True   d) False   e) False

As asthma is now frequently diagnosed before the age of 2 and sometimes even before the age of 1, signs suggestive of an alternative diagnosis must be remembered. Asthma at all ages gives a polyphonic wheeze. An inhaled foreign body and vascular ring give a monophonic wheeze. Cystic fibrosis and aspiration pneumonia have polyphonic wheeze.

207   a) False   b) False   c) False   d) True   e) True

Migratory polyarthralgia is characteristic of rheumatic fever. The platelet count in Henoch–Schönlein purpura is normal. Joint damage is not permanent.

208   a) True   b) True   c) True   d) True   e) False

The value of a tick-box approach for developmental screening is now being questioned. Thus such checklists are not included in the Personal Child Health Records.

209   a) True   b) False   c) False   d) False   e) True

210   a) True   b) False   c) True   d) True   e) True

Pulmonary blood flow is decreased in tricuspid atresia.

211   a) False   b) True   c) True   d) True   e) True

None of the sons of an affected male is affected, unless the mother is a carrier or is also affected. Half of the offspring of an affected male and a female carrier will manifest the condition, with a quarter being homozygously affected females and a quarter being affected males. Lyon's hypothesis is that only one X-chromosome is active in each cell, and the number of 'active', abnormal Xs a carrier has determines the extent of her showing any signs of the condition.

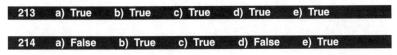

212 **a) True** **b) False** **c) True** **d) True** **e) False**

Croup (laryngotracheobronchitis) causes upper airway obstruction and should be distinguishable from asthma. Tuberculosis, though rarer in developed countries, is a possible differential diagnosis. Moreover, early chemotherapy and control measures are important because of the appearance of multiple drug-resistant strains. Anaphylactic attacks may cause both upper and lower airway obstruction. However, the acute nature should be distinguishable from asthma.

213 **a) True** **b) True** **c) True** **d) True** **e) True**

214 **a) False** **b) True** **c) True** **d) False** **e) True**

In eczema herpeticum, herpes type 2 is also possible, e.g. in child sexual abuse cases.

215 **a) True** **b) False** **c) False** **d) False** **e) False**

216 **a) True** **b) True** **c) False** **d) False** **e) False**

Children with special educational needs should be educated in normal schools if possible. The arrangement has to be in the best interest of the child with special needs and his peers.

217 **a) True** **b) False** **c) True** **d) False** **e) True**

Hepatitis A is transmissible by anal-oral contact in heterosexuals and in homosexuals. For children, 720 ELISA units should be given. For unimmunized contact cases, human normal immunoglobulin and hepatitis A vaccine are given. Immunization should theoretically be offered to all whose sexual behaviour is likely to put them at risk.

218 **a) True** **b) True** **c) True** **d) False** **e) True**

219 **a) True** **b) True** **c) True** **d) False** **e) True**

220 **a) True** **b) True** **c) False** **d) True** **e) False**

Live vaccines are contraindicated 3 weeks before and 3 months after an immunoglobulin injection. Two live vaccines can be given simultaneously to two sites which are far apart. Otherwise, they should be given at least 3 weeks apart.

221   a) True   b) True   c) False   d) False   e) False

The examiner should exert gentle upward force on the child's mastoid processes. The child should be looking forward. The standard deviation of the measurements should be no more than 0.3 cm.

222   a) False   b) False   c) False   d) False   e) False

He is now totally protected from hepatitis B but his HBsAb titre is expected to fall later. The titre should thus be checked 5 years later. If it is between 10–100 miu/ml, 1 booster injection is given. If it is more than 100 miu/ml, his HBsAb should be checked after a further 5 years. If the HBsAb is below 10 miu/ml, which is unlikely to be the case, the whole course of vaccination might need to be repeated.

223   a) False   b) False   c) True   d) False   e) False

224   a) False   b) False   c) True   d) False   e) False

Most children can walk upstairs with 2 feet per step at 21 months. Most can build a tower of 6 to 8 bricks, turn door knobs and turn pages singly at 2 years.

225   a) True   b) False   c) True   d) False   e) False

Most children can walk on tiptoe, after demonstration, at $2\frac{1}{2}$ years. Most can ride a tricycle and unbutton large buttons at 3 years.

226   a) False   b) True   c) False   d) True   e) True

Most babies have hand-hand transfer at 6 months. Most have pincer grasp for small objects at 10 months. At 18 months, most can feed themselves with a cup, though with some spillage.

227   a) False   b) True   c) True   d) False   e) False

The Sheldon Report (1967) recommended that child health services in the community be provided by general practitioners.

228   a) True   b) True   c) True   d) True   e) True

In general, any live viral vaccine, viral infection or immunosuppressive state may cause false negative tuberculin results.

229   a) False   b) True   c) False   d) False   e) True

The step-care plan is currently recommended by the National Asthma Campaign. Step 1 is the occasional use of inhaled bronchodilators when required. Step 3 is the regular, prophylactic use of low dose, inhaled steroids. Step 4 is the regular use of higher dose inhaled steroids. A child may commence treatment at any step and later be stepped up or down. Regular review is essential. A similar plan of management is available for adult asthma and guidelines are available for the management of acute asthma attacks in children and adults.

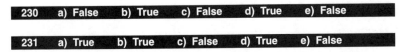

230	a) False	b) True	c) False	d) True	e) False

231	a) True	b) True	c) False	d) True	e) False

In the present scheme, two doses of MMR are given at 12 to 15 months and 3 to 5 years. Td (a low dose of diphtheria) is given at 13 to 18 years. Only three doses of Hib are given, at 2, 3 and 4 months. Hepatitis B vaccine is not routinely given in the UK.

232	a) True	b) True	c) True	d) True	e) True

In Bernard–Soulier disease, there are large platelets with decreased glycoprotein Ib. It is a congenital disorder of platelet function. The other important congenital cause is von Willebrand's disease. Uraemia, aspirin, dysproteinaemia and cardiopulmonary bypass are all acquired disorders of platelet function.

233	a) False	b) False	c) False	d) True	e) False

This is a case of secondary enuresis. A secondary cause is likely to be present and the cause should be identified before any therapeutic and behavioural intervention.

234	a) True	b) False	c) True	d) False	e) False

Arthralgia and thrombocytopenia are complications of rubella. Measles and chicken pox might lead to pneumonia.

235	a) True	b) False	c) True	d) False	e) True

Most children can copy a square and button up large buttons at 4 years.

236	a) True	b) False	c) True	d) False	e) True

A pulse rate of more than 140/min and respiration of more than 50 breaths/min are indicative of a severe asthma attack.

237	a) True	b) False	c) False	d) False	e) True

Treatment can be started at the step most appropriate to the initial severity and frequency of asthma attacks. Systemic steroids, used as a rescue course, are totally acceptable, no matter at which step the child is currently receiving treatment.

238	a) False	b) False	c) True	d) False	e) True

The endogenous eczemas are: atopic eczema, seborrhoeic dermatitis (dermatitis = eczema), pompholyx, gravitational eczema, asteatotic eczema and discoid eczema. The exogenous eczemas are: irritant contact dermatitis, allergic contact dermatitis and photocontact dermatitis. Not all are seen in children.

| 239 | a) False | b) True | c) False | d) False | e) True |

| 240 | a) False | b) False | c) True | d) False | e) True |

The incubation periods for measles, glandular fever (due to EBV) and mumps are 10 to 14 days, 1 to 8 weeks and 14 to 21 days respectively.

241 In facial nerve palsy:

a) Bell's palsy causes a lower motor neuron lesion
b) Cerebral palsy causes an upper motor neuron lesion
c) Ramsay–Hunt syndrome causes an upper motor neuron lesion
d) A history of hypertension can be relevant
e) Only the lower half of the face is affected in upper motor neuron lesions

242 Particular problems in the management of chronic asthma in children below the age of 2 include:

a) Family history is usually absent
b) Diagnosis is based entirely on investigations
c) Poor compliance of parents
d) Bronchodilators are not effective below the age of 1
e) Many other conditions mimic asthma at this age

243 Duties of the district nurse might include:

a) Dressings for injuries
b) Education for mothers in the child health clinics
c) Immunization
d) Liaison with the night nursing services
e) Measuring the growth parameters

244 Causes of conjugated neonatal hyperbilirubinaemia include:

a) Hypothyroidism
b) Pyloric stenosis
c) G6PD deficiency
d) Congenital cytomegalovirus infection
e) Congenital hepatitis B

245 Causes of proximal renal tubular acidosis are:

a) Renal tubular necrosis
b) Phenacetin
c) Chronic renal failure
d) Hyperparathyroidism
e) Nephrotic syndrome

246 The following diseases can now be diagnosed prenatally:

a) Phenylketonuria
b) Homocystinuria
c) Severe combined immunodeficiency
d) Fanconi's anaemia
e) Lesch–Nyhan syndrome

247 An operation may be indicated for tongue tie if:

a) The child has dysarthria at the age of 3
b) The tie is thick and approaches the tip of the tongue at birth
c) The child cannot lick his upper lip
d) The palatal arch is high
e) The parents are distressed about the tie and request an operation

248 A 15-year-old boy has sudden onset of right testicular pain. Examination reveals tender, non-swollen, high-lying right testis. The most likely diagnosis is:

a) Haematocele
b) Torsion of testis
c) Strangulated inguinal hernia
d) Testicular neoplasm
e) Acute epididymitis

249 An 18-month-old girl presents with rose-pink papules on the trunk and neck on the fourth day of fever.

a) Measles is unlikely if MMR vaccination was given at 12 to 15 months
b) Strict isolation is not needed
c) The fever is expected to continue for 4 more days
d) Ataxia is a likely complication
e) Rubella is the likely diagnosis if the MMR vaccine was missed

250 A pink newborn with a heart rate of 88/min is actively gasping. He has good muscle tone and responds to nasal catheter stimulation with facial grimace. The Apgar score is:

a) 5
b) 6
c) 7
d) 8
e) 9

251 Causes of bow legs include:

a) Trauma
b) Normal variation
c) Rickets
d) Blount's disease
e) Poliomyelitis

252 Management approaches for squint include:

a) Orthoptic exercises
b) Occluding the squinting eye
c) Surgery to shorten the left medial rectus for a left convergent squint
d) Surgery to lengthen the left lateral rectus for a right divergent squint.
e) Spectacles to correct refractive errors

253 **Investigations which can safely be performed in a day-care setting are:**

a) Sweat test
b) Oral glucose tolerance test
c) Suprapubic tap for urine
d) Intravenous urogram
e) Micturating cystourethrogram

254 **Examples of good parenting include:**

a) Ignoring the child when he is having a temper tantrum
b) Setting structures and routines in daily life
c) Setting clear limits for behaviour
d) Avoiding love and affection if a child has recurrent breath holding attacks
e) Giving rewards if the child eats well

255 **Giant hairy naevi:**

a) Are called 'bathing trunk naevi' if very large
b) Are not premalignant
c) Are abnormalities of dermal melanocytes
d) The parents should be safely reassured
e) Might need surgical removal with skin grafting

256 **The following congenital heart diseases are unlikely to present at birth:**

a) Hypoplastic left heart
b) Truncus arteriosus
c) Endocardial fibroelastosis
d) Severe aortic stenosis
e) Total anomalous pulmonary venous drainage

257 **Of congenital HIV infection:**

a) The risk of affecting the baby in developed countries is about 50%
b) The risk is not affected by antiviral therapy
c) Breast feeding should be discouraged in developed countries
d) HIV Ab is useful for early diagnosis
e) P24 antigen and polymerase chain reaction are helpful in early diagnosis

258 **The following statements are true:**

a) Audit is an example of quality assurance activities
b) The major types of audit include that of structure, process and outcome
c) Audit allows a more effective use of time and energy
d) Audit is a valuable educational tool
e) An example of audit is to study whether influenza vaccine can lower the exacerbation of attacks in children with asthma

259   Duties of the district nurse might include:

a) Venepuncture
b) Social support
c) Ear syringing
d) Surveillance of children at risk of abuse
e) Wound management

260   Problems of a child with cerebral palsy include:

a) Vision problems
b) Muscle contractures
c) Cocktail party speech
d) Hearing impairment
e) Lack of primitive reflexes

261   For the hypersensitivities:

a) IgE is implicated in type I (anaphylactic) responses
b) Contact dermatitis is a good example of type I response
c) Rhesus and ABO iso-immunization are due to type II (cytotoxic) responses
d) Henoch–Schönlein purpura is an example of type III (circulating immune complexes) responses
e) Hay fever is an example of type IV (cell mediated or delayed) response

262   The Reynell Developmental Language Scale:

a) Caters for children aged 1 to 10
b) Detects dysarthria
c) Assesses verbal comprehension and verbal expression
d) Has been validly and reliably translated to languages other than English
e) Can safely be used by general practitioners for screening purposes

263   Child abuse should be suspected if there are:

a) Explanations for the injuries which do not match the appearance of the injuries
b) A single injury
c) Classic abuse appearances
d) Immediate presentation of injury
e) Injuries in older children

264   Tricyclic antidepressant poisoning causes:

a) Ataxia
b) Abnormal postures
c) Arrhythmia
d) Agitation
e) Anticholinergic effects

265 Normal gross motor development is as follows:

a) 6 weeks: momentary neck extension in ventral suspension
b) 10 weeks: head well extended in ventral suspension
c) 4 months: spontaneously elevates the head when supine
d) 6 months: sits steadily with no need for any support
e) 9 months: walks with one hand held

266 Causes of ptosis include:

a) Horner syndrome
b) Crouzon's disease
c) Fetal alcohol syndrome
d) Aarsog syndrome
e) Apert syndrome

267 In atrial septal defect:

a) The primum type is associated with mitral regurgitation
b) The secundum type typically presents late
c) Reduced exercise tolerance is characteristic
d) Central cyanosis in the newborn period is characteristic
e) No treatment is indicated if asymptomatic

268 In hypochromic anaemia:

a) Serum ferritin is decreased in iron deficiency
b) Total iron binding capacity is decreased in iron deficiency
c) Serum ferritin is normal in thalassaemia
d) Total iron binding capacity is markedly increased in thalassaemia
e) Serum ferritin is decreased in anaemias due to chronic infection

269 Influenza vaccine:

a) Contains one type A and two type B sub-types
b) Is prepared each year with strains considered most likely to be prevalent the following winter
c) Gives virtually 100% protection
d) Is indicated for children with asthma
e) Is contraindicated if the eczema of a child is thought to be exacerbated by eggs

270 The following are target groups for BCG vaccination:

a) School children aged 10 to 14
b) Infants whose parents request for BCG
c) Contacts of cases of active pulmonary tuberculosis
d) Tuberculin positive children
e) Children from countries with a high prevalence of tuberculosis

271 In phenylketonuria:

a) The blood phenylalanine level should be monitored weekly in the initial phase of treatment
b) Blood phenylalanine levels in the range of 484–1210 μmol/l is acceptable
c) A system of '50 mg phe exchanges' exists where the total daily allowance of milk is fixed
d) Refined carbohydrates are restricted
e) Cheese and eggs should be encouraged

272 In-toeing may be caused by:

a) Femoral anteversion
b) Sitting in the 'television position'
c) Metatarsus vulgus
d) Femoral retroversion
e) Medial tibial torsion

273 Complications of pertussis include:

a) Bronchiectasis
b) Intracranial haemorrhage
c) Encephalitis
d) Failure to thrive
e) Peripheral neuritis

274 For a clumsy child, the following conditions should be ruled out:

a) Drug effects
b) Spinal muscular atrophy
c) Ataxia telangiectasia
d) Cerebellar ataxia
e) Cerebral palsy

275 Iatrogenic causes of growth suppression include:

a) Inhaled steroids at 200 μg/day
b) Inhaled steroids at 400 μg/day
c) Systemic steroids
d) Cranial irradiation
e) Spinal irradiation

276 In foster care:

a) Long term fostering usually involves young children
b) Short term fostering should not extend beyond 2 years
c) The usual limit to the number of foster children is three
d) Allowances are paid to the foster parents
e) Private fostering is illegal

277 **Management for children with beta-thalassaemia major includes:**

a) Hypertransfusion scheme
b) Iron and folate supplements
c) Management of diabetes mellitus
d) Desferrioxamine
e) Genetic counselling

278 **Jaundice on day 1 is often caused by:**

a) Metabolic disorders
b) TORCHS infections
c) Gastrointestinal obstruction
d) Haemolysis
e) Physiological factors

279 **Children with epilepsy should not:**

a) Ride a bicycle on the open road
b) Swim when supervised
c) Climb ropes
d) Inform their teachers about the epilepsy
e) Study in a normal school

280 **Cleft lip:**

a) Occurs more frequently in females
b) Is associated with trisomy 13
c) Is associated with a history of epilepsy of the mother
d) May lead to language delay
e) May lead to abnormal dentition

281 **Edward syndrome is associated with:**

a) Trisomy 13
b) Trisomy hands
c) Long sternum
d) Prominent occiput
e) Survival rate of 80% at 1 year

282 **The following are compatible with prerenal failure:**

a) Urine/plasma urea ratio less than 4 : 1
b) Urine osmolality 300 mmol/kg
c) Urine osmolality 450 mmol/kg
d) Sunken eyes
e) Increased urine output after saline infusion

283 The following are contraindications to at least some vaccines:

a) History of neonatal jaundice
b) Failure to thrive
c) On replacement steroids
d) On systemic antibiotics
e) Cerebral palsy

284 The following are common causes of neonatal thrombocytopenia:

a) Maternal anti-platelet antibodies
b) Infection
c) Hyperglycinaemia
d) Asphyxia
e) Leukaemia

285 In cystic fibrosis:

a) Fat restriction is essential because of malabsorption and steatorrhoea
b) Pancreatic enzyme replacements are essential
c) Fat soluble vitamins are supplemented
d) Diet supplements are needed in periods of illness
e) Overnight tube feeding is an option

286 Characteristic features of classical migraine are:

a) Duration of days
b) Aura
c) Hemiplegia
d) Photophobia
e) Sudden pain around one eye

287 Problems of babies born to mothers with poorly controlled diabetes mellitus include:

a) Hypermagnesaemia
b) Polycythaemia
c) Hypocalcaemia
d) Sacral agenesis
e) Respiratory distress

288 Epidemiology of asthma:

a) About 200 to 300 children die each year from asthma in England and Wales
b) There is a steady decrease in mortality rate in the 5 to 14 year-old age group
c) There is no change in mortality rate in the 0 to 4 year-old age age group
d) The point prevalence of asthma is increasing
e) The point prevalence of atopic eczema is increasing

289 The following statements are true:

a) Gaiters are usually used to prevent extension contractures of the arm
b) A standing frame can prevent flexion contractures of the hips
c) Non-slip bathmats prevent slip-and-fall injuries
d) Bean-bags prevent rigidity in a spastic child
e) Wedges can assist a hypotonic child to have head and spinal control

290 A full term infant has tachypnoea with grunting. Chest X-ray shows well expanded lungs with streaky shadows radiating from the bilateral hilar regions. The most likely diagnosis is:

a) Transient tachypnoea of the newborn
b) Congenital pneumonia
c) Bronchopulmonary dysplasia
d) Meconium aspiration
e) Aspiration pneumonia

291 Anal signs of sexual abuse include:

a) Reflex anal dilatation
b) Anal fissures
c) Anal skin tags
d) Tyre sign
e) Perianal bruising

292 Advantages of special schools include:

a) Expert teachers
b) Normal expectations
c) Larger classes
d) Health service support
e) Provision of transport

293 The following are target groups for BCG vaccination:

a) Children whose parents request for BCG
b) Infants from countries with a high prevalence of tuberculosis
c) HIV-positive children
d) Children with frequent episodic asthma
e) Children who will stay in Africa for more than 1 month

294 When taken by a breastfeeding mother:

a) Sulphonamides cause neonatal jaundice
b) Indomethacin causes the grey baby syndrome
c) Augmentin causes convulsions in the baby
d) Benzodiazepines cause hypotonia in the baby
e) Lithium causes hyperthermia of the baby

295 **In anorexia nervosa:**

a) The patient may come from a family with a medical or paramedical background
b) A distorted body image is characteristic
c) There is loss of 20% of previous body weight
d) The patient should be persuaded to transfer the responsibility of weight gain to the doctor
e) Primary amenorrhoea can be present

296 **Head-banging:**

a) Can occur during sleep
b) Is a manifestation of insecurity
c) Virtually all stops at the age of 4
d) Is associated with cataracts
e) Is a type of spasmus nutans

297 **The following conditions can cause an acute loss of vision:**

a) Migraine
b) Cataracts
c) Hysteria
d) Niemann–Pick disease
e) Epilepsy

298 **The following statements are true:**

a) Virtually 100% of 4-year-olds have retractable prepuce
b) 20% of infants have undescended testes at birth
c) Operations for maldescended testes do not decrease the risk of malignancy
d) All inguinal hernias do not transilluminate
e) Enlargement of the clitoris is compatible with normality in the newborn

299 **In atrioventricular canal defect:**

a) Heart failure in the first few weeks is likely
b) Failure to thrive is characteristic
c) Pulses are usually normal
d) Cardiomegaly is usual
e) Incomplete right bundle branch block is usual

300 **In epidemiology:**

a) Prevalence takes into account the chronicity of the condition
b) Incidence is often used to monitor chronic conditions
c) The stillbirth rate is the number of babies born dead with a gestational age of at least 28 weeks per 100 total births
d) The neonatal mortality rate is the number of babies who die in the first 30 days of life per 1000 live births
e) The infant mortality rate is the number of infants who die in the first 12 months of life per 1000 total births

241   a) True   b) True   c) False   d) True   e) True

Ramsay–Hunt syndrome is a herpes zoster infection along the facial nerve. It is a lower motor neuron lesion.

242   a) True   b) False   c) True   d) False   e) True

There is usually no family history of atopy or asthma. The diagnosis is based almost entirely on symptoms and signs, rather than objective lung function tests. It is very difficult to persuade parents that asthma does present at such an age, particularly if there is no objective test and no family history. The response to inhaled bronchodilators is variable. Foreign bodies, cystic fibrosis, reflux and congenital abnormalities are among the other conditions which are differential diagnoses of asthma at this age.

243   a) True   b) False   c) True   d) True   e) True

Education for the parents in the child health clinic is more properly the responsibility of the health visitor.

244   a) False   b) False   c) False   d) True   e) True

245   a) False   b) False   c) False   d) True   e) True

246   a) True   b) True   c) True   d) True   e) True

247   a) False   b) False   c) True   d) False   e) False

A thick tongue tie approaching the tip of the tongue is common for many normal infants. That the child cannot lick his upper lip is an indication that the tie is severe. If there are symptoms, an operation may be justified.

248   a) False   b) True   c) False   d) False   e) False

249   a) True   b) True   c) False   d) False   e) False

The child is most likely to be suffering from roseola infantum. This is due to human herpes virus type 6 and probably type 7 infection. The fever typically subsides on the same day as the rash appears. Rubella presents with day 1 rash.

250   a) False   b) False   c) False   d) True   e) False

251   a) True   b) True   c) True   d) True   e) False

Blount's disease is osteochondritis of the upper medial aspect of tibia. Poliomyelitis usually leads to knock knees.

252   a) True   b) False   c) False   d) False   e) True

The good eye should be occluded instead of the squinting eye. For a left convergent squint, the left medial rectus should be lengthened or the left lateral rectus shortened. For a left lateral squint, the right medial rectus should be shortened or the right lateral rectus lengthened. Surgery is generally performed for cosmetic indications.

253   a) True   b) True   c) True   d) True   e) True

254   a) True   b) True   c) True   d) False   e) False

Reasonable discipline is needed. This must be accompanied by love, or it fails. Whether a child can finish his plate or not, no bribes or punishment should be given. Eating is an enjoyment for the child and he should not be praised or scolded.

255   a) True   b) False   c) True   d) False   e) True

25–30% of all giant hairy naevi will undergo malignant change. Thus, many would advise on surgical treatment. Otherwise, very close observation with clinical photographs is needed.

256   a) False   b) False   c) False   d) False   e) False

All these congenital heart diseases can present at days after birth.

257   a) False   b) False   c) True   d) False   e) True

In developed countries, without antiviral treatment, about 15–20% of infants born to HIV positive mothers will finally be infected. It is now well documented that reverse transcriptase inhibitors given in pregnancy lower the risk. Whether urease inhibitors should be added remains to be seen. HIV Ab is not useful for early diagnosis because of maternal transmission of antibodies.

258   a) True   b) True   c) True   d) True   e) False

To study whether a vaccine is effective or not should be regarded as a research activity rather than audit. An audit activity in such a context may be to evaluate the uptake of the vaccine and the major factors limiting the uptake.

259   a) True   b) True   c) True   d) False   e) True

Surveillance of children at risk of abuse is one of the duties of the health visitor.

260   a) True   b) True   c) False   d) True   e) False

'Cocktail party' speech is characteristic of children with spina bifida. It is the persistence of primitive reflexes which is a problem in cerebral palsy.

261   a) True   b) False   c) True   d) True   e) False

Contact dermatitis is an example of type IV (cell-mediated or delayed) response. Hay fever is a typical type I (anaphylactic) response.

262   a) False   b) False   c) True   d) True   e) False

The Reynell Developmental Language Scale caters for children from 6 months to 6 years of age. Scores are given for verbal comprehension and verbal expression, and an overall score with age equivalence is also available. Dysarthria is not assessed. The test should not be lightly undertaken for screening by general practitioners as the child will learn in the process and will not give a valid score when formally tested by specialists in the child development clinic later.

263   a) True   b) False   c) True   d) False   e) False

Multiple injuries, delayed presentation and injuries of young and very young children should lead to a suspicion of non-accidental injury.

264   a) True   b) True   c) True   d) True   e) True

These are the five **A**s in TCA poisoning. The treatment is to manage the **a**cidosis and **a**rrhythmia and consider giving **a**nticholinesterase.

265   a) True   b) True   c) False   d) False   e) False

Most children can elevate the head spontaneously when lying supine at 6 months, sit steadily without support at 8 to 9 months and walk with one hand held at 1 year.

266   a) True   b) False   c) True   d) True   e) True

All three commoner syndromes of craniosynostosis (Apert's, Carpenter's and Crouzon's) can have proptosis, but proptosis is most prominent in Crouzon's syndrome. Pstosis is related to third nerve palsy due to pressure effect, and is commonly seen only in Apert's syndrome. See standard textbooks for other features.

267   a) True   b) True   c) True   d) False   e) False

There is no central cyanosis in the neonatal period for ASD as there is no right-to-left shunt. Surgical closure is indicated to prevent heart failure, pulmonary hypertension and arrhythmia.

268   a) True   b) False   c) False   d) False   e) False

The total iron binding capacity is increased in iron deficiency. Serum ferritin is markedly increased in thalassaemias. Total iron binding capacity is usually normal in thalassaemias. The serum ferritin is usually increased in anaemias due to chronic infection.

269 **a) False** **b) True** **c) False** **d) True** **e) False**

Influenza vaccine consists of two type As and one type B subtypes. As the strains are constantly changing due to antigenic drifts and shifts, yearly injections are needed. The protection rate is 70–80%. It is indicated for children with chronic respiratory disease, chronic heart disease, chronic renal failure, diabetes mellitus or immunosuppression. It is contraindicated in persons with a known anaphylactic reaction to eggs and egg products.

270 **a) True** **b) True** **c) True** **d) False** **e) True**

A positive tuberculin result is a contraindication for BCG vaccination.

271 **a) False** **b) False** **c) False** **d) False** **e) False**

The blood phenylalanine level should be monitored daily in the initial phase of treatment. The acceptable range is 120–350 µmol/l. Phe can be provided by foods other than milk. Thus, the total daily allowance of phe is fixed and foods are given in '50 mg phe exchanges'. Refined carbohydrates are freely allowed and cheese and eggs are totally restricted.

272 **a) True** **b) True** **c) False** **d) False** **e) True**

The 'television position' is sitting with knees touching each other, knees fully flexed and hips medially rotated. Such a posture is said to enhance in-toeing formation. The child should therefore be advised to sit in the 'Buddha' position with knees flexed and hips abducted and externally rotated. Metatarsus varus is a cause of in-toeing, not metatarsus vulgus.

273 **a) True** **b) True** **c) True** **d) True** **e) True**

274 **a) True** **b) True** **c) True** **d) True** **e) True**

Drugs such as anticonvulsants may cause ataxia leading to clumsiness.

275 **a) False** **b) False** **c) True** **d) True** **e) True**

Inhaled steroids at doses of more than 800 µg/day might lead to HPA axis suppression.

276 **a) False** **b) False** **c) True** **d) True** **e) False**

Long-term fostering usually involves older children, as young children should best be adopted. Short-term fostering should not extend beyond 6 months. Private arrangements for fostering are legal. The local authority is required to visit to ensure that the foster parents are suitable.

277   a) True   b) False   c) True   d) True   e) True

Children with beta-thalassaemia major already have iron overload and iron supplements are thus not needed. The desferrioxamine is given by a subcutaneous pump.

278   a) False   b) True   c) False   d) True   e) False

279   a) True   b) False   c) True   d) False   e) False

The teachers must be informed explicitly. They should be taught how to deal with a fit in the school. If they know the half-truth, unnecessary restrictions might be placed on the child.

280   a) False   b) True   c) True   d) True   e) True

The male: female ratio for cleft lip is about 2:1. Cleft lip is associated with Patau's syndrome and phenytoin syndrome. The language delay is related to dysarthria and frequent otitis media.

281   a) False   b) True   c) False   d) True   e) False

Edward syndrome is trisomy 18. Trisomy 13 is Patau's syndrome. Infants with Edward syndrome have a short sternum and a less than 10% survival rate to 1 year.

282   a) False   b) False   c) True   d) True   e) True

A low urine/plasma urea ratio and a low urine osmolality are seen in intrarenal and postrenal failure. Sunken eyes are a sign of dehydration, which is associated with prerenal failure.

283   a) False   b) False   c) False   d) False   e) False

These are all false contraindications to immunizations.

284   a) False   b) True   c) False   d) True   e) False

Maternal anti-platelet antibodies is an uncommon cause of neonatal thrombocytopenia. Hyperglycinaemia and leukaemia are rare causes.

285   a) False   b) True   c) True   d) True   e) True

Fat intake is now recommended to be normal or high with enzyme replacement therapy.

286   a) False   b) True   c) False   d) True   e) False

A duration of days suggests common migraine rather than classical migraine. Hemiplegia is suggestive of hemiplegic migraine and sudden pain around one eye is characteristic of cluster migraine.

287   a) False   b) True   c) True   d) True   e) True

Hypomagnesaemia is an associated feature.

288   a) False   b) False   c) False   d) True   e) True

About 40 to 45 children die each year from asthma in England and Wales. There is no change in the mortality rate in the 5–14-year-old age group. A steady decrease is noted in the mortality rate in the 0–4-year-old age group.

289   a) False   b) True   c) True   d) False   e) True

Gaiters are mainly used to prevent flexion contractures. Bean-bags are contraindicated in a spastic child as they enhance the formation of wind-swept deformities.

290   a) True   b) False   c) False   d) False   e) False

291   a) True   b) True   c) False   d) True   e) True

It must be remembered that all such signs, especially reflex anal dilatation, are not pathognomonic of child sexual abuse. The tyre sign is said to be present when there is perianal oedema.

292   a) True   b) False   c) False   d) True   e) True

Special schools have smaller classes and this is an advantage.

293   a) True   b) True   c) False   d) False   e) True

HIV positivity is a contraindication while frequent episodic asthma is not an indication.

294   a) True   b) False   c) False   d) True   e) False

It is chloramphenicol which causes the grey baby syndrome. Lithium in breast milk may lead to hypothermia.

295   a) True   b) True   c) False   d) False   e) True

There is a loss of 20% of the expected body weight relative to the height, not 20% of the previous body weight. The patient should be encouraged to take responsibility for the recovery. Both primary and secondary amenorrhoea can occur in anorexia nervosa.

296   a) True   b) True   c) False   d) True   e) False

Head banging can persist into the school years.

297 a) True   b) False   c) True   d) False   e) True

Cataracts and Niemann–Pick disease cause progressive loss of vision.

298 a) False   b) False   c) True   d) False   e) True

About 85–90% of 4-year-olds have retractable prepuces. About 3% of infants have undescended testes at birth. Operations do not decrease the risk of malignant change in maldescended testes. However, they do make malignancy easier and earlier to detect. Inguinal hernias in children frequently do transilluminate. Some enlargement of the clitoris at birth is normal. Excessive enlargement should, of course, lead to suspicions of congenital adrenal hyperplasia.

299 a) True   b) True   c) True   d) True   e) True

300 a) True   b) False   c) False   d) False   e) False

Incidence is used to monitor acute conditions. At present, a cut-off line of 24 weeks is being used for stillbirth in view of the improved perinatal care for premature infants. The neonatal mortality rate is the number of babies dying in the first 28 days of life per 1000 live births. The infant mortality rate is the number of infants dying in the first 12 months of life per 1000 live births.

301 Injuries characteristic of child abuse are:

a) Mongolian spot
b) Torn frenulum
c) Petechial haemorrhage on the face
d) Striae
e) Cheek bruises

302 Teething can cause:

a) Fever
b) Diarrhoea
c) Irritability
d) Convulsions
e) Excessive salivation

303 The following statements are true:

a) The deviation changes in concomitant squint
b) The deviation depends on the direction of gaze in inconcomitant squint
c) In alternating squint, the squint alternates between a convergent and a divergent squint
d) When performing the cover test, the eye being covered is being tested
e) When performing an uncover test, inconcomitant manifest squint is tested

304 Risk factors for child abuse include:

a) More than 18 months between birth of children
b) History of parents having been abused as children
c) Unemployment
d) Mother aged 21 or above
e) Low birth-weight infant

305 Recognised causes of chronic diarrhoea include:

a) Wiskott–Aldrich syndrome
b) Kawasaki disease
c) Zollinger–Ellison syndrome
d) Haemolytic-uraemic syndrome
e) Di George's syndrome

306 Management for children with beta-thalassaemia major might include:

a) Psychosocial support
b) Splenectomy
c) Analgesics for painful crises
d) Bone marrow transplantation
e) Management of delayed puberty

307 In salicylate poisoning:

a) Metabolic acidosis is common
b) Respiratory acidosis is common
c) Respiratory alkalosis is common
d) If the serum salicylate level is 30 mg/dl 4 hours after ingestion, the child should be safely sent home
e) Alkaline diuresis is indicated if the serum salicylate level is 80 mg/dl

308 A 6-week-old infant has recurrent attacks of projectile vomiting after normal feeding. He is dehydrated and constipated. The most likely diagnosis is:

a) Pyloric stenosis
b) Hiatus hernia
c) Duodenal atresia
d) Diaphragmatic hernia
e) Hirschsprung's disease

309 Reference Standard

	+ve	−ve
New Test +ve	a	b
New Test −ve	c	d

a) Sensitivity of the new test = $\dfrac{a}{a+b}$
b) Specificity of the new test = $\dfrac{d}{c+d}$
c) Positive predictive value of the new test = $\dfrac{a}{a+c}$
d) Yield of the new test = $\dfrac{a}{a+b+c}$
e) Incremental yield of the new test = $\dfrac{a}{a+b+c+d}$

310 The following statements are true:

a) Slow weight gain is a presentation of urinary tract infection (UTI)
b) Bed wetting is a presentation of UTI
c) Symptoms of UTI are non-specific for children under the age of 2
d) More than half of the children with dysuria and frequency have UTI
e) It is rare for small girls to have vulvovaginitis

311 Common causes of raised intracranial pressure are:

a) Intracranial haemorrhage
b) Meningitis
c) Benign intracranial hypertension
d) Encephalitis
e) Reye's syndrome

312 **In an immunization clinic:**

a) A general practitioner is usually conducting the interviews
b) Up-to-date ampoules of 1 : 1000 adrenaline must be kept
c) Written consent for immunization is often obtained
d) The current health of the child is checked
e) Mothers are warned about the side effects of the vaccines

313 **The following conditions signify diseases in the newborn:**

a) Peeling of skin of the hands and feet
b) Blanched on one side of the body and pink on the opposite side
c) Pinhead lesions on the nose
d) Peripheral cyanosis
e) Oedema of one arm

314 **Successful legislation has led to a decrease in the following types of accidents:**

a) Car passenger injuries
b) House fires
c) Burns
d) Insect bites
e) Playground injuries

315 **Programmes on accident prevention should emphasize:**

a) The acquisition of accurate local information
b) Education for small children
c) Education for the parents
d) Participation of the public
e) Teaching of first-aid

316 **For the oral rehydration solutions (ORS):**

a) WHO-ORS contain 35 mmol/l of sodium
b) WHO-ORS contain 20 mmol/l of potassium
c) WHO-ORS are suitable for use in developed countries
d) Commercially available ORS have 90 mmol/l of sodium
e) Anti-diarrhoeal agents should be administered concomitantly

317 **For the ethnic groups:**

a) Sikhs do not eat beef
b) Hindus do not eat dairy products
c) Hindus are mostly vegetarians
d) Moslems do not eat beef
e) Moslems are mostly vegetarians

93

318 **A child has uncorrected visual acuity (VA) of 4/60 in the right eye and 6/30 in the left eye. He has corrected VA of 6/24 in the right eye and 40/60 in the left eye:**

a) His right eye is considered blind
b) His right eye is considered partially sighted
c) His left eye is considered partially sighted
d) He is partially sighted
e) He is not partially sighted

319 **Sexual abuse should be suspected when:**

a) There is sexual behaviour inappropriate for age
b) Behavioural problems exist
c) The child is caught in masturbation
d) The child discloses the facts
e) Sexually transmitted diseases are diagnosed

320 **The following statements are true:**

a) A disability is a loss or abnormality of anatomical structures or physiological functions
b) Ambloypia is a disability
c) A handicap is a restriction in performing an activity in a manner considered normal for a human being
d) The inability to see the blackboard clearly is an example of a handicap
e) Tertiary preventive activities decrease disabilities and handicaps

321 **Principles in a child health promotion programme include:**

a) A partnership with parents
b) An aim to increase the confidence of the parents
c) Team work
d) The general practitioner is the major health professional for child health promotion for pre-school children
e) The paediatrician is the major health professional for child health promotion for school children

322 **For schoolchildren and teenagers:**

a) Three different kinds of fruits and vegetables should be consumed daily
b) Semi-skimmed milk is unacceptable
c) Cheese and yoghurt may replace milk
d) Fats should be allowed to be eaten until the child has had enough
e) Two helpings of meat daily is recommended

323 **According to the 1986 Education Act:**

a) A 'Statement of Special Needs' should be drafted for children with learning difficulties
b) Children with special needs should be educated in ordinary schools if possible
c) School governors have the responsibility of deciding whether sex education should be part of the curriculum or not
d) Parents' views should be respected in regard to sex education in the school
e) Parents have a legal right to withdraw their children from school sex education

324 **A 2$\frac{1}{2}$-year-old child is having temper tantrums because his mother refuses to buy him a toy car. His mother should:**

a) Buy him the toy car
b) Punish him immediately by non-corporal means
c) Ignore him
d) Praise him when he stops crying
e) Scold him when he stops crying

325 **For Munchausen syndrome by proxy:**

a) The carer genuinely believes that the child is ill
b) The carer may contaminate the child's urine or stool samples
c) The child's life is never in danger
d) The diagnosis should be considered only when convincing evidence is present
e) It is a cause of sudden infant death

326 **Indications of the pneumococcal vaccine include:**

a) HIV infection
b) Frequent pneumonia
c) Sickle cell disease
d) Diabetes mellitus
e) History of pneumococcal meningitis

327 **The aims of a child health service are:**

a) To provide a high quality health service to all children
b) To screen for congenital abnormalities according to the requests of the parents
c) To support families in the care of their children
d) To promote a safe and healthy environment for children
e) To encourage parents to depend on professionals as much as possible

328 A 10-month-old girl has been in close contact with a cousin with measles. She is seen 2 days after the exposure:

a) Nothing should be done now as she will receive the MMR vaccine at 12 to 15 months
b) She should be given MMR vaccine now
c) She should be given dilute immunoglobulin
d) She should be given MMR vaccine together with dilute immunoglobulin now
e) She should be given MMR vaccine together with concentrated immunoglobulin now

329 Growth hormone deficiency:

a) Is more common in boys
b) Leads to delayed bone age
c) Leads to little or no rise in the growth hormone level in challenge tests
d) Is a spectrum of diseases
e) Is treated by human growth hormone produced by DNA recombinant technology

330 The following association of dietary restrictions are true:

a) Hindu and beef
b) Sikh and pork
c) Muslim and pork
d) Buddhist and meat
e) Jewish and beef

331 Köebner phenomenon is demonstrated in:

a) Pityriasis versicolor
b) Viral warts
c) Pityriasis rosea
d) Tinea corporis
e) Lichen planus

332 In a child with asthma, the following features suggest an alternative diagnosis:

a) Absence of family history
b) Chronic infection
c) Absence of other atopic features
d) Vomiting with choking
e) Monophonic wheeze

333 Clinitest is positive in:

a) Galactosaemia
b) Diabetes mellitus
c) Fructosaemia
d) Lactosuria
e) Normal infants

334 A baby reacts to every minor stimulus with a moro reflex. The knee and ankle jerks are brisk. Ankle clonus is demonstrable. She is feeding well with normal growth parameters. The serum glucose and calcium levels are normal. The most likely diagnosis is:

a) Pyridoxine dependency
b) Meningitis
c) Intraventricular haemorrhage
d) Cerebral palsy
e) Normal

335 It is recommended that:

a) A neonatal physical examination should be performed for every baby routinely
b) A 6 to 8 week review should be undertaken
c) The blood pressure of every neonate should be checked
d) The school entrant medical examination should be continued
e) Microurinalysis at the school entrant examination should not be justified as a good screening test

336 Specific immunoglobulins are available for:

a) Hepatitis A
b) Diphtheria
c) Pertussis
d) Tetanus
e) Hepatitis B

337 The following are compatible with acute pharyngitis:

a) Facial erythematous rash with perioral pallor
b) Fever with rose spots on day 7
c) Palatal petechiae
d) Greyish-white membrane covering the pharynx
e) Discrete white nodules with surrounding erythema on the cheek mucosa

338 Methods to screen for hearing impairment in the newborn include:

a) Oto-acoustic emissions
b) Acoustic response cradle
c) Distraction testing
d) STYCAR tests
e) Auditory brainstem evoked responses

339 Advice to a family with a history of sudden infant death includes:

a) Stop smoking in the house
b) Install apnoea alarm
c) Learn resuscitation techniques for babies
d) Encourage formula feeding
e) Avoiding overheating for babies

340 The following features favour a diagnosis of cystic fibrosis rather than untreated coeliac disease:

a) Meconium ileus
b) Failure to thrive
c) Poor appetite
d) Frequent chest infections
e) Delayed puberty

341 For the pure tone audiometry:

a) Frequencies from 500–4000 Hz are generally tested
b) Consonants occupy a narrower range of frequencies than vowels
c) The minimum age that can be tested is 6 years
d) A large discrepancy between air and bone conduction signifies sensorineural hearing loss
e) A child with hearing impairment at 40 dB will have difficulty in following normal speech

342 Children of teenage mothers are at risk from:

a) Child abuse
b) Poor academic performance
c) Accidents
d) Intrauterine growth retardation
e) Delayed language development

343 Advice to a family with a history of sudden infant death includes:

a) Do not let babies sleep prone
b) Avoid overlaying
c) Encourage breastfeeding
d) Babies should not be swaddled tightly in blankets
e) Use baby duvets

344 The following statements are true:

a) Positive HBcAb (anti-HBc) signifies a history of natural infection
b) A child immunized against hepatitis B successfully will have HBsAb positive and HBcAb negative
c) Negative HBsAg and negative HBsAb signify that the child has not been in any contact with hepatitis B
d) Positive HBeAg and negative HBeAb signify high infectivity
e) Positive HBsAg, negative HBsAb, negative HBeAg and negative HBeAb signify that the child is not having active infection

345 A 4-month-old infant has recurrent episodes of pneumonia. He is irritable during feeds with frequent large volume vomits. Blood picture reveals hypochromic microcytic anaemia. The most likely diagnosis is:

a) Excessive tea drinking
b) Pyloric stenosis
c) Cystic fibrosis
d) Hiatus hernia
e) Choanal atresia

346 Babies born to mothers with the following hepatitis status should be given both hepatitis B vaccination and immunoglobulin:

a) HBsAg +ve, HBeAg +ve, HBeAb –ve
b) HBsAg –ve, HBsAb –ve, IgM anti-HBc +ve
c) HBsAg –ve, HBsAb +ve, total anti-HBc –ve
d) HBsAg +ve, HBeAgAb unknown
e) HBsAg +ve, HBeAg –ve, HBeAb +ve

347 The following can give rise to a concomitant squint:

a) Retinoblastoma
b) Corneal opacity
c) Cataract
d) Cerebral palsy
e) Meningitis

348 The following are causes of sensorineural hearing loss:

a) Congenital cytomegalovirus infection
b) Serous otitis media
c) Usher's syndrome
d) Gentamicin
e) Ear wax

349 Screening methods to detect congenital dislocation of the hips might include:

a) A checklist for the risk factors
b) The Ortolani–Barlow manoeuvre
c) Observation for limited abduction and asymmetric skin creases
d) Observation for gait abnormality
e) Ultrasound scanning

350 The following associations are true:

a) Atopic eczema and a poorly-defined border
b) Seborrhoeic eczema and a well-defined border
c) Discoid eczema and a well-defined border
d) Irritant contact dermatitis and a well-defined border
e) Pompholyx and a poorly-defined border

351 In a child with asthma, the following features suggest an alternative diagnosis:

a) Focal lung signs
b) Prominent nocturnal symptoms
c) Cardiovascular signs
d) Failure to thrive
e) Not exacerbated by exercise

352 The following statements regarding the Hib vaccine are true:

a) It is a capsular polysaccharide
b) It can be safely mixed with the DPT vaccines
c) Children under 13 months should receive 3 injections
d) Unimmunized children 13 to 48 months should receive 3 injections
e) Children aged 4 and above should receive 1 injection if they have not been immunized

353 Growing pains:

a) Occur at periods of maximum growth
b) Are due to differences in growth velocities of bones and tendons
c) Occur predominantly at 4 to 8 years
d) Are associated with osteosarcoma
e) Are associated with the periodic syndrome

354 A 10-month-old girl has been in close contact with a cousin with mumps. She is seen 72 hours after the exposure:

a) Nothing should be done now. Give the MMR routinely at 12 to 15 months
b) She should be given the MMR vaccine now
c) She should be given mumps-specific immunoglobulin
d) She should be given MMR vaccine together with mump-specific immunoglobulin
e) She should be given MMR vaccine together with human normal immunoglobulin

355 In complete heart block in children:

a) The heart rate is absolutely regular with no change on exercising
b) The block is always persistent
c) Adam–Stokes' attacks are rare in children
d) Extreme bradycardia is an indication for a pacemaker
e) Heart failure in young infants is an indication for a pacemaker

356 The following therapeutic associations are true:

a) ACTH and infantile spasm
b) Valproate and myoclonic seizures
c) Clonazepam and infantile spasm
d) Vigabactrin and infantile spasm
e) Phenytoin and febrile convulsions

357 A child has extensive second degree burn. Management includes:

a) Adequate analgesia
b) Adequate hydration
c) Maintenance of patent airway
d) Antitetanus prophylaxis
e) Antibiotic prophylaxis

358 The following are characteristic of transposition of great arteries:

a) Central cyanosis
b) Soft, muffled, second heart sound
c) Ejection systolic murmur
d) Chest X-ray showing boot-shaped heart
e) Plethoric lung fields

359 Babies born to mothers with the following hepatitis serological status should be given hepatitis B immunoglobulin:

a) HBsAg –ve, IgM anti-HBc +ve (4 weeks before delivery)
b) HBsAg –ve, IgM anti-HBc –ve, HBsAb +ve, total anti-HBc +ve
c) HBsAg +ve, HBeAg +ve, HBeAb –ve
d) HBsAg +ve, HBeAgAb unknown
e) HBsAg +ve, HBeAg –ve, HBeAb +ve

360 A 5-year-old girl has been in close contact with another child who has developed meningitis. It is diagnosed to be *Neisseria meningitidis* serogroup C. The girl is seen 2 days after the contact.

a) Nothing can be done for her now
b) She should be given meningococcal A + C vaccine only
c) She should be given immunoglobulin only
d) She should be given meningococcal A+C vaccine with rifampicin now
e) She should be given meningococcal A+C vaccine with immunoglobulin now

301 a) False b) True c) True d) False e) True

Petechial haemorrhages on the face may signify strangulation, although other causes are possible, e.g. pertussis. Striae are due to obesity, pubertal growth or Cushing's syndrome.

302 a) False b) False c) True d) False e) True

That teething can cause fever and diarrhoea is wrongly believed by many parents.

303 a) False b) True c) False d) False e) False

The deviation is constant in concomitant squint. When performing the cover test, the uncovered eye is being tested. The uncover test is to detect a latent squint.

304 a) False b) True c) True d) False e) True

Children less than 18 months old and mothers less than 20 years old are at a higher risk for child abuse.

305 a) True b) False c) True d) False e) True

Kawasaki disease and haemolytic uraemic syndrome are associated with acute diarrhoea.

306 a) True b) True c) False d) True e) True

Splenectomy is indicated for some cases, when the need for transfusion is especially high. Painful crises occur in sickle cell disease.

307 a) True b) False c) False d) True e) True

Respiratory acidosis is not associated. Respiratory alkalosis is associated as salicylates are respiratory stimulants. It is however relatively uncommon. A serum salicylate level of 45 mg/dl in the first 6 hours is safe.

308 a) True b) False c) False d) False e) False

309 a) False b) False c) False d) False e) False

The sensitivity is $a/(a+c)$. The specificity is $d/(b+d)$. The positive predictive value is $a/(a+b)$. The yield is $a/(a+b+c+d)$.

The incremental yield of a new test = yield of the new test – yield of the old test, e.g.

	Reference Standard	
	+ve	–ve
New Test +ve	a	b
–ve	c	d

	Reference Standard	
	+ve	–ve
Old Test +ve	a'	b'
–ve	c'	d'

The incremental yield =

$$\frac{a}{a+b+c+d} - \frac{a'}{a+b+c+d}$$

310   a) True   b) True   c) True   d) False   e) False

Only about 20% of all children with dysuria and frequency really have urinary tract infection. Thus it is important to document the infection before treatment. Vulvovaginitis is, in fact, very common as a differential diagnosis of urinary tract infection. Most are not related to sexual abuse or *Enterobius vermicularis* infestation.

311   a) True   b) True   c) False   d) True   e) True

Benign intracranial hypertension and Reye's syndrome are rare causes.

312   a) False   b) True   c) False   d) True   e) True

The running of an immunization clinic is usually conducted by the health visitor. Up-to-date adrenaline ampoules must be kept in case of anaphylactic reactions. The bringing of a child for immunization implies informed consent. Thus, written consent is usually not necessary. The health status of the child is checked to make sure that there is no contraindication for immunization.

313   a) False   b) False   c) False   d) False   e) False

Peeling of the hands and feet, peripheral cyanosis and oedema of one arm are all physiological in the newborn period. Harlequin colour change, the blanching of one side of the body with pink colour on the other side, is not uncommonly seen. Pinhead lesions on the nose are milia.

314   a) True   b) True   c) True   d) False   e) True

Legislation has led to the compulsory use of suitable seat belts and carriage seats for infants and children, the use of flame-proof fabrics and better design of playground facilities.

315   a) True   b) False   c) True   d) True   e) True

Education for small children is not effective. Education for older children and parents, and the modification of the environment, are far more effective.

316   a) False   b) True   c) False   d) False   e) False

WHO-ORS contain 90 mmol/l sodium. It is suitable for use in developing countries. Commercially available ORS has 35 mmol/l sodium and is designed for use in developed countries. Anti-diarrhoeal agents slow the transit time in the gut and might encourage the formation of an abnormal flora in the gut.

317   a) True   b) False   c) True   d) False   e) False

Moslems do not eat pork. Most of them are not vegetarians as they usually eat chicken or mutton.

103

318 a) False b) False c) False d) False e) True

'Partially sighted' refers to a person and not an eye. A person with corrected VA of 4/60 to 6/24 in the better eye is partially sighted. A person with corrected VA of 3/60 or worse in the better eye should be registered as 'blind'.

319 a) True b) True c) False d) True e) True

Masturbation is normal behaviour and should not lead to a suspicion of sexual abuse.

320 a) False b) False c) False d) False e) True

An impairment is a loss or abnormality of an anatomical structure of a physiological function. A disability is a restriction in performing an activity in a manner considered normal for a human being. A handicap is the failure to fulfil a vocational task or to play a suitable role in the society. Tertiary preventive activities decrease disabilities and handicaps by preventing the development of complications.

321 a) True b) True c) True d) False e) False

Empowerment is to increase the confidence of the parents and to minimize unnecessary dependence on professionals. The health visitor is the major professional for child health promotion for pre-school children. The school nurse is the major health professional for child health promotion for school children.

322 a) False b) True c) True d) False e) True

Five different kinds of fruits and vegetables should be consumed daily. Semi-skimmed milk is acceptable for children over 5 years of age. Cereals, not fats, should be allowed to be eaten until the child has had enough.

323 a) False b) False c) True d) True e) False

'Special needs' and 'Statements of Special Needs' are covered in the 1981 Education Act.

324 a) False b) False c) True d) False e) False

The boy should neither be punished nor rewarded. He should be ignored so as to give him negative reinforcement for his attention-seeking behaviour. However, once he stops crying, there should not be prolonged disapproval. He should be treated as if nothing has happened. The mother may try to reason with him later, not during the tantrum or immediately after the tantrum.

325 a) False b) True c) False d) False e) True

A very high index of suspicion is needed to diagnose Munchausen syndrome by proxy, which is now considered a form of child abuse. Thus, the evidence should be actively sought. It is a cause of sudden infant death, although the exact proportion might never be known.

326   a) True   b) False   c) True   d) True   e) False

All stages of HIV infections are indications for the pneumococcal vaccine. For frequent pneumonia the underlying cause should first be identified. In sickle cell disease, autosplenectomy occurs and thus the pneumococcal vaccine is indicated.

327   a) True   b) False   c) True   d) True   e) False

Screening procedures should fulfil Wilson's criteria and many other considerations, including cost-effectiveness and resources in the community. Empowerment of the parents should be encouraged, rather than unnecessary dependence on professionals.

328   a) False   b) True   c) False   d) False   e) False

Immunoglobulin might attenuate the immune response to rubella and mumps and should not be given. MMR should be given now and repeated later. MMR is useful for post-exposure prophylaxis against measles but not against rubella and mumps as the immune responses against rubella and mumps are too slow to be of any immediate use.

329   a) True   b) True   c) True   d) True   e) True

Growth hormone deficiency is a spectrum of diseases from absolute deficiency to borderline normal cases. With DNA recombinant technology there is now no danger of the slow viral encephalopathies.

330   a) True   b) False   c) True   d) True   e) False

Sikhs do not eat beef. Jews do not eat pork. Almost all meats are restricted for the Buddhists.

331   a) False   b) True   c) False   d) False   e) True

The lesions of viral warts, lichen planus and psoriasis appear in the sites of previous trauma.

332   a) False   b) True   c) False   d) True   e) True

333   a) True   b) True   c) True   d) True   e) False

Clinitest detects any reducing sugar and clinistix detects glucose only. Thus, galactosaemia, fructosaemia and lactosuria have clinitest +ve and clinistix –ve, diabetes mellitus has clinitest +ve and clinistix +ve, and normal infants have clinitest –ve and clinistix –ve.

334   a) False   b) False   c) False   d) False   e) True

The diagnosis is a jittery baby within the normal range.

335	a) True	b) True	c) False	d) True	e) True

336	a) False	b) False	c) False	d) True	e) True

Four types of specific immunoglobulins are available, against tetanus, hepatitis B, rabies and varicella-zoster respectively. For other diseases, if immunoglobulins are indicated, normal human immunoglobulin is given.

337	a) True	b) True	c) True	d) True	e) True

Facial erythematous rash with perioral pallor is compatible with scarlet fever with pharyngitis. Pharyngitis in typhoid might have rose rash on day 7. Pharyngitis in infectious mononucleosis might have palatal petechiae. Pharyngitis in diphtheria might have a greyish-white membrane covering the pharynx. Discrete white nodules on the cheek mucosa with surrounding erythema are Koplik spots. They appear on day 2 in a child suffering from measles with pharyngitis.

338	a) True	b) True	c) False	d) False	e) True

339	a) True	b) True	c) True	d) False	e) True

An apnoea alarm, although not of proven benefit, may be helpful psychologically for the parents. Breastfeeding should be encouraged.

340	a) True	b) False	c) False	d) True	e) False

Failure to thrive and delayed puberty occur in both cystic fibrosis and coeliac disease. Poor appetite is a feature of coeliac disease. Children with cystic fibrosis have good appetites.

341	a) True	b) False	c) False	d) False	e) True

Consonants occupy a wider range of frequencies. 'T' and 'S' may be missed by a child with high-tone hearing impairment. Most children at 4 years can reliably be tested. A large discrepancy between air and bone conduction signifies conductive hearing loss.

342	a) True	b) True	c) True	d) True	e) True

343	a) True	b) True	c) True	d) True	e) False

344	a) True	b) True	c) False	d) True	e) False

For most cases, HBsAg –ve and HBsAb –ve signify that the child has not been in contact with hepatitis B. However, the child might well be in the 'window period' just after an acute hepatitis infection. He can have HBsAg –ve, HBsAb –ve, total anti-HBc +ve and IgM anti-HBc +ve. His HBsAb may thus become positive later. HBeAg +ve and HBeAb –ve signify high infectivity and the infant of a mother with such a serological status should be given vaccination and immunoglobulin. HBsAg +ve, HBsAb –ve, ve, HBeAg –ve and HBe Ab –ve do not signify that the person is not having active infection. Only HBsAg +ve, HBsAb –ve, HBeAg –ve and HBeAb +ve do. This is because 'e mutants' are present and might give a false negative result to traditional HBeAg tests. In such a case, hepatitis B DNA by polymerase chain reaction should be checked.

345   a) False   b) False   c) False   d) True   e) False

The baby has hiatus hernia with gastro-oesophageal reflux.

346   a) True   b) True   c) False   d) True   e) False

A mother with HBsAg –ve, HBsAb –ve and IgM anti-HBc +ve has acute hepatitis. She is in the 'window period' now. The baby should be given both hepatitis B vaccine and immunoglobulin at birth. A mother with HBsAg –ve, HBsAb +ve and total anti-HBc –ve has been successfully vaccinated against hepatitis B. Nothing should be done for the baby. The mother with HBsAg +ve with HBeAgAb unknown might have HBeAg +ve. If the results cannot be immediately available it is safer to give both hepatitis B vaccine and immunoglobulin to the baby at birth. For the mother with HBsAg +ve, HBeAg –ve and HBeAb +ve, the infectivity is low. The current guidelines recommend that only vaccination is to be given, not immunoglobulin.

347   a) True   b) True   c) True   d) True   e) True

All such cases can affect the visual pathway from the cornea to the visual cortex and give a concomitant squint.

348   a) True   b) False   c) True   d) True   e) False

349   a) True   b) True   c) True   d) True   e) True

Using a checklist is the simplest screening method for many conditions. Ultrasound screening might be feasible, although the incremental yield and cost-effectiveness are yet to be determined.

350   a) True   b) False   c) True   d) False   e) True

The borders of seborrhoeic dermatitis and irritant contact dermatitis are usually not well-defined.

351   a) True   b) False   c) True   d) True   e) False

352   a) True   b) True   c) True   d) False   e) False

Invasive diseases are caused by encapsulated forms. According to the recommendations of the manufacturers, Hib and DPT vaccines can be safely mixed (for some combinations). Children under 13 months should receive three injections, 1 month apart for each. Unimmunized children 13 to 48 months old should receive only a single injection. Vaccination for children over 4 is not needed as the incidence of invasive Hib disease is very low after 4 years.

353   a) False   b) False   c) False   d) False   e) True

Growing pains occur most predominantly at 8 to 12 years. Children with growing pains have more recurrent abdominal pains and headaches.

354   a) True   b) False   c) False   d) False   e) False

The development of immunity is too slow for post-exposure vaccination to be of any use in mumps.

355   a) False   b) False   c) False   d) True   e) True

Complete heart block in children can be intermittent. Unlike in adults, the heart rate is not absolutely fixed.

356   a) True   b) True   c) True   d) True   e) False

There is no need for any prophylactic medication for febrile convulsions.

357   a) True   b) True   c) True   d) True   e) True

358   a) True   b) False   c) False   d) False   e) True

The second heart sound is loud and single. No murmur is present. The heart looks like an 'egg lying on its side' on the chest X-ray.

359   a) True   b) False   c) True   d) True   e) False

The mother with HBsAg –ve and IgM anti-HBc +ve had acute hepatitis B during pregnancy. The baby should receive both hepatitis B vaccination and immunoglobulin at birth. If the mother has HBsAg –ve, HBsAb +ve, IgM anti-HBc –ve and total anti-HBc +ve, no immunoglobulin should be given unless there is a history of acute hepatitis in the pregnancy. Babies born to mothers with HBsAg +ve, HBeAg +ve and HBeAb –ve; or HBsAg +ve with HBeAgAb unknown; should receive both vaccination and immunoglobulin. Immunoglobulin does not need to be given to babies whose mothers have HBsAg +ve, HBeAg –ve and HBeAb +ve. However, hepatitis B vaccine should still be given.

360   a) False   b) False   c) False   d) True   e) False

361 The following are recognised as sexually transmissible diseases:

a) Hepatitis A
b) Hepatitis B
c) Hepatitis C
d) Delta hepatitis
e) Hepatitis E

362 The procedures in audit are:

(1) Examining the changes necessary
(2) Measuring the performance
(3) Closing the audit loop
(4) Comparing the performance with the standard
The correct sequence is:

a) (4), (1), (2), (3)
b) (4), (2), (1), (3)
c) (2), (1), (3), (4)
d) (2), (4), (1), (3)
e) (2), (1), (4), (3)

363 Prothrombin time is increased in:

a) Factor VII deficiency
b) Haemophilia B
c) Factor X deficiency
d) Haemophilia A
e) Von Willebrand's disease

364 The external criteria for the Dubowitz score for gestational age include:

a) Breast size
b) Skin texture
c) External genitalia
d) Lanugo hairs
e) Nose firmness

365 Wilson and Jungner's criteria for screening programmes include the following:

a) The test should have high sensitivity and specificity
b) The test should be cost-effective
c) The condition should be important
d) The condition should be a congenital condition
e) A latent or asymptomatic stage should be present

366 The following statements are true:

a) Colour vision testing should be part of the pre-school examination
b) Colour vision problems are much more common in boys than in girls
c) The Ishihara test consists of a series of five dots in a crucifix pattern
d) The City University Plates test consists of plates of small circles with a hidden number or curve
e) Tritanopia is very rare

367 HIV positive children can receive the following vaccines:

a) BCG
b) MMR
c) DPT
d) Inactivated polio
e) Hepatitis B

368 Diseases caused by *Haemophilus influenzae* include:

a) Pneumonia
b) Pericarditis
c) Osteomyelitis
d) Septic arthritis
e) Septicaemia

369 The following associations regarding the Heaf test are true:

a) Grade 0 — give BCG if not already received in the past
b) Grade 1 — give BCG if not already received in the past
c) Grade 2 — no further action
d) Grade 3 — refer to chest clinic, prophylactic chemotherapy may be needed
e) Grade 4 — refer to chest clinic, prophylactic chemotherapy may be needed

370 The following are associated with an increased risk of congenital dislocation of the hips:

a) Breech presentation
b) Male sex
c) Postural deformities of the feet
d) Family history of congenital dislocation of hips
e) Polyhydramnios

371 A cephalohaematoma:

a) Must be differentiated from a subperiosteal haemorrhage
b) Is usually visible at birth
c) May calcify
d) May be associated with underlying fracture of the skull
e) Should be managed surgically

372 **The following conditions should be routinely screened for all children:**

a) Neuroblastoma
b) Urinary tract infection
c) Liver disease in infancy
d) Familial hypercholesterolaemia
e) Phenylketonuria

373 **Disadvantages of formula feeding include:**

a) Underfeeding
b) Infection
c) Haemorrhagic disease of the newborn
d) Electrolyte disorders
e) Cows' milk protein intolerance

374 **The yield of a screening test can be improved by:**

a) Increasing the sensitivity
b) Increasing the specificity
c) Repeating the test for test-negative cases
d) Repeating the test for test-positive cases
e) Screening only the high risk groups

375 **Beta thalassaemia is common in:**

a) Northern China
b) Asia minor
c) India
d) Italy
e) South-east Asia

376 **The following statements are true:**

a) The normal infant is myopic
b) Distant vision is not impaired in hypermetropia
c) Congenital myopia is associated with retinal detachment
d) Myopia is corrected with convex lenses
e) Retinoscopy detects the visual acuity in young children

377 **Drug effects on the fetus:**

a) Isotretinion can lead to CNS defects, mainly if given in the third trimester
b) Phenytoin can lead to cleft lip, finger and toe abnormalities, mainly if given in the second trimester
c) Carbimazole causes goitre, mainly if given in the third trimester
d) Warfarin can lead to neonatal haemorrhage, mainly if given in the first trimester
e) Valproate can lead to neural tube defects, mainly if given in the third trimester

378 **Regarding impetigo contagiosa:**

a) The bullous form is usually caused by Streptococci
b) The non-bullous form is usually caused by Staphylococci
c) Psoriasis is a usual predisposing factor
d) The golden crusts can be removed gently
e) The bullous form is usually caused by beta-lactamase-producing strains

379 **The following statements are true:**

a) The total number of adoptions in England and Wales has been continually falling since 1974
b) The average age of adopted children is slowly rising
c) Better support for single parents is an important factor in the decline of number of adoptions
d) Two people applying to adopt together must be married
e) Adopted people have the right of access to their original birth certificates on reaching the age of 18

380 **For a newborn:**

a) Both eyes should be inspected routinely
b) Fundoscopy should be performed routinely
c) The red reflex should be examined routinely
d) The eye examination should be repeated at 6 to 8 weeks routinely
e) The eye examination should be repeated at 18 to 24 months routinely

381 **The following recommendations regarding the storage of vaccines are true:**

a) Vaccines should be stored in the storage compartments of the refrigerator door
b) Food and drinks must not be stored in the refrigerator used to store vaccines
c) When vaccines are despatched by post, they should not be accepted if 72 hours have elapsed since posting
d) Refrigerators should be defrosted regularly
e) Domestic refrigerators are generally adequate for vaccine storage

382 **In growth monitoring:**

a) The length of every neonate should be measured routinely
b) The length measurement should be repeated routinely at 6 to 8 weeks and 6 to 9 months
c) The height should be measured at 18 to 24 months routinely
d) The weight should be measured at 6 to 8 weeks, 6 to 9 months and 18 to 24 months routinely
e) Facilities should be provided for the parents to weigh the babies themselves

383 **Common cold (coryza) is caused by:**

a) Adenovirus
b) Rhinovirus
c) Respiratory syncytial virus
d) Rotavirus
e) Parainfluenza virus

384 **In a normal (Gaussian) distribution:**

a) The mean is at the 50th percentile
b) About 95% of all values lie between –3 SD and +3 SD
c) About 70% of all values lie between –2 SD and +2 SD
d) Prepubertal height follows such a distribution closely
e) Prepubertal weight follows such a distribution closely

385 **Measures to reduce bicycle accidents include:**

a) Doubling
b) Reflective aids at night
c) Helmets
d) Suitably sized bicycles
e) Bright clothes by day

386 **A 1-year-old child can:**

a) Scribble spontaneously
b) Kiss on request
c) Build a tower of 3 bricks
d) Turn pages singly
e) Walk with one arm held

387 **The following are compatible with intrarenal or postrenal failure:**

a) Urine osmolality 250 mmol/kg
b) Urine osmolality 300 mmol/kg
c) Marked diuresis after relief of the obstruction
d) Urine/plasma urea ratio more than 4:1
e) No response in urine output after saline infusion

388 **The following statements are true:**

a) Screening for hypertension is not justifiable at present (for children)
b) Screening for asthma is not justifiable at present
c) The testes should be examined at birth and at 6 to 8 weeks
d) The testicular examination should be repeated at 18 to 24 months
e) The number of boys with untreated, undescended testes over 5 years can be an indicator of the success of the screening programme

389 **Cyanotic congenital heart diseases in the newborn include:**

a) Transposition of great arteries
b) Pulmonary stenosis
c) Fallot's tetralogy
d) Ventricular septal defect
e) Tricuspid atresia.

390 **The following diseases are notifiable:**

a) Mumps
b) Viral hepatitis
c) Malaria
d) Rubella
e) AIDS

391 **In asthma management:**

a) An 18-month-old child can use a valved spacer with a face mask
b) A 2-year-old child can use a metered dose inhaler with a valved spacer
c) A 3-year-old child can use powder inhalers
d) A 7-year-old child is too old to use a metered dose inhaler with a valved spacer
e) A 10-year-old child can use a metered dose inhaler on its own

392 **The following rashes are typically pruritic:**

a) Pityriasis rosea
b) Pityriasis versicolor
c) Papular urticaria
d) Pityriasis alba
e) Nodular prurigo

393 **The following diseases are notifiable:**

a) HIV infection
b) Amoebic dysentery
c) Measles
d) Acute encephalitis
e) Tuberculosis

394 **The following conditions produce a pendular nystagmus:**

a) Benign positional vertigo
b) Severe refractive errors of the eye
c) Intracranial tumour
d) Cataract
e) Phenytoin

395 The following statements are true:

a) Distant vision is best tested at 10 feet
b) Single letters are preferable to linear charts in vision testing
c) Diagrams can replace letters for testing vision in small children
d) Both the corrected and uncorrected visual acuities should be determined
e) Near vision is tested at 50 cm

396 Viral warts:

a) Are caused by human papilloma viruses
b) Will not resolve if left untreated
c) On the faces of children should be treated with electrocautery
d) Can be completely cured by keratolytic agents
e) Should not be treated with cryosurgery for children

397 A 7-month-old boy has been in close contact with another child with rubella. He is seen 1 day after the exposure:

a) Nothing should be done now. Give the MMR vaccine at 12 to 15 months
b) He should receive MMR vaccine only now
c) He should receive MMR vaccine together with rubella-specific immunoglobulin now
d) He should receive MMR vaccine together with human normal immunoglobulin now
e) He should receive human normal immunoglobulin only now

398 Causes of projectile vomiting include:

a) Duodenal ulcer
b) Raised intracranial pressure
c) Pyloric stenosis
d) Gastroenteritis
e) Urinary tract infection

399 The following congenital disorders require immediate (within the first week) treatment after birth:

a) Haemangioma
b) Imperforated anus
c) Choanal atresia
d) Hypospadias
e) Congenital diaphragmatic hernia

400 The following favour a diagnosis of nephroblastoma rather than neuroblastoma:

a) Age of 4 years
b) Does not cross midline of abdomen
c) Pallor with weight loss
d) Calcifications seen in ultrasound
e) Metastases to lung

401 The following statements relating to the case conference in suspected child abuse are true:

a) It is usually held during the period covered by the Emergency Protection Order
b) Full biographies of the parents and carers are essential
c) Decisions are usually made by simple majority vote
d) The decision to put the child on the Child Protection Register is usually made by the consultant paediatrician in charge of the child
e) Parents and carers have no right to attend

402 The following medications can be safely taken while breastfeeding:

a) Thyroxin
b) Antacids
c) Theophylline
d) Chlorpheniramine
e) Carbimazole

403 For children with migraine:

a) About 50% have a family history of migraine
b) Stress in schoolwork is a frequent exacerbating factor
c) Attacks may be precipitated by cheese or cherries
d) Attacks may be precipitated by physical exercise
e) Attacks may be precipitated in the premenstrual period

404 The case conference in suspected child abuse might be attended by:

a) Ward sister
b) Police
c) Parents
d) Probation officer
e) General practitioner

405 The following are associated with dysarthria:

a) Myotonic dystrophy
b) Down's syndrome
c) Cerebral palsy
d) Beckwith's syndrome
e) Tongue tie

406 Causes of irregular hepatosplenomegaly are:

a) Polycystic disease of the liver
b) Sickle cell disease
c) Macronodular cirrhosis
d) Lymphoma
e) Harmatoma

407 Predisposing factors for iron deficiency are:

a) Prematurity
b) Beta-thalassaemia major
c) Infestation
d) Giving cows' milk before the age of 1
e) Tea drinking

408 Vulvovaginal signs of sexual abuse include:

a) Scarring of the vaginal wall
b) Clitoromegaly
c) Hymenal tears
d) Attenuated hymen
e) Tearing of the posterior fourchette

409 A child of short stature is referred for investigation. The height of his father is 167 cm and that of his mother is 149 cm:

a) The mid-parental height is 158 cm
b) The mid-parental height is 166 cm
c) The expected range of the final height of the child is 156 to 172 cm
d) The expected range of the final height of the child is 154 to 162 cm
e) The expected range cannot be determined without knowledge of the present age and height of the child

410 A 6-year-old child has frequent headaches. Indications for referral are:

a) Change in behaviour
b) Headaches exacerbated by psychological stress
c) Headaches precipitated by chocolate and cherries
d) Abnormal neurological signs
e) Headaches aggravated by coughing

411 Babies born to mothers with the following hepatitis serological status should be given hepatitis B vaccine:

a) HBsAg +ve, HBeAg −ve, HBeAb +ve
b) HBsAg −ve, HBsAb +ve, total anti-HBc −ve
c) HBsAg +ve, HBeAgAb unknown, total anti-HBc +ve
d) HBsAg +ve, HBeAg +ve, HBeAb −ve
e) HBsAg −ve, IgM anti-HBc +ve (5 weeks before delivery), total anti-HBc +ve

412 Causes of unconjugated neonatal hyperbilirubinaemia include:

a) Alpha-1-antitrypsin deficiency
b) Galactossaemia
c) Pyloric stenosis
d) ABO incompatibility
e) Gilbert syndrome

413 Characteristics of febrile convulsions include:

a) Onset before 6 months
b) Duration of less than 20 minutes
c) No focal or atypical features
d) Associated with rapid rising phase of fever
e) Associated with CNS infections

414 Causes of a positive sweat test (sodium of 70 mmol/l or more) include:

a) Cushing's syndrome
b) Nephrogenic diabetes insipidus
c) Cystic fibrosis
d) Thyrotoxicosis
e) Ectodermal dysplasia

415 In growth monitoring:

a) The head circumference should be routinely measured before discharge from hospital for every newborn
b) The head circumference measurement should be repeated at 6 to 8 weeks routinely for every infant
c) If the head circumference is crossing the centiles upwards with signs suggestive of hydrocephalus, the measurement should be repeated over several months to consider whether referral is needed
d) If the head circumference is crossing the centiles upwards with no signs suggestive of hydrocephalus, the measurement should be repeated over several months to consider whether referral is needed
e) If the head circumference is crossing the centiles downwards and the baby is well and thriving, the parents should be informed that the baby might be abnormal

416 Common causes of epistaxis in children include:

a) Trauma
b) Bleeding disorders
c) Infection
d) Foreign bodies
e) Tumour

417 For a child with pyrexia of unknown origin:

a) An undiagnosed bacterial infection is most likely
b) Connective tissue disorders account for less than 1% of cases
c) Up to 50% will remain undiagnosed
d) Munchausen syndrome by proxy should not be suspected unless overwhelming evidence is present
e) Kawasaki disease is a possible diagnosis

418 The following are appropriate dosages for children:

a) Phenytoin 100 mg/kg/24 h orally
b) Benzylpenicillin 50 mg/kg/24 h intramuscularly
c) Carbamazepine 75 mg/kg/24 h orally
d) Ampicillin 250 mg/kg/24 h orally
e) Paracetamol 250 mg/kg/24 h orally

419 The following statements are true:

a) Breast milk contains 80% casein and 20% whey
b) IgA is mainly present in the whey protein
c) The average infant will require 110 ml of milk per kg body weight per day
d) Bottle-fed infants should be fed on demand
e) It is clearly shown that casein-based formulae are more satisfying

420 Characteristic findings in a preterm baby include:

a) Chin reaching only to tip of shoulder
b) Full wrist flexion
c) Flat on couch when lying prone
d) Incomplete ankle dorsiflexion
e) Incomplete knee extension with hips fully flexed

361   a) True   b) True   c) True   d) False   e) False

Hepatitis A can be transmitted by oral-anal contact in heterosexuals and homosexuals. Sexual transmission for hepatitis C is well established. However, the risk is relatively low. Sex as a route for transmission of delta hepatitis and hepatitis E is not yet established.

362   a) False   b) False   c) False   d) True   e) False

363   a) True   b) False   c) True   d) False   e) False

The extrinsic pathway is affected in factor VII deficiency. The intrinsic pathway is affected for haemophilia A and B. Both pathways are affected in factor X deficiency. Von Willebrand's disease is mainly a disorder of platelet aggregation.

364   a) True   b) True   c) True   d) True   e) False

365   a) True   b) True   c) True   d) False   e) True

366   a) False   b) True   c) False   d) False   e) True

There is no evidence to justify routine screening for colour vision defects in the pre-school examination. A series of five dots in a crucifix pattern is the City University Plates test. The subject decides which of the four peripheral dots best matches the colour of the central dot. The Ishihara test consists of plates of small circles with a hidden number or path for the subject to identify.

367   a) False   b) True   c) True   d) True   e) True

HIV positivity is a contraindication for BCG, as there is a danger of disseminated BCG infection. That MMR vaccine is a live vaccine is not a contraindication in HIV-infected children. Inactivated polio (Salk) can be used instead of oral polio (Sabin) vaccine.

368   a) True   b) True   c) True   d) True   e) True

369   a) True   b) True   c) True   d) True   e) True

No further action needs to be taken for a grade 2 reaction if it is a routine testing for asymptomatic children.

370   a) True   b) False ·   c) True   d) True   e) False

Female sex and oligohydramnios are risk factors.

371   a) False   b) False   c) True   d) True   e) False

Cephalohaematoma is a subperiosteal haemorrhage. It is usually visible, at the earliest, hours after birth. Surgical treatment is unnecessary and may lead to infection and haemorrhage. Almost all resolve spontaneously, though some may become bony prominences later.

372   a) False   b) False   c) False   d) False   e) True

Familial hypercholesterolaemia should be screened for only if there is a family history.

373   a) False   b) True   c) False   d) True   e) True

Underfeeding is uncommon as the amount consumed is obvious to the mother. Haemorrhagic disease of the newborn almost never occurs in formula-fed babies.

374   a) True   b) False   c) True   d) False   e) True

Increasing the specificity might decrease the number of false positive cases. However, the number of true positives may also be decreased and thus the yield is usually decreased. Test positive cases should be referred for confirmative testing. The same test should not be repeated.

375   a) False   b) True   c) True   d) True   e) True

376   a) False   b) False   c) True   d) False   e) False

The normal infant is hypermetropic. Myopia is corrected by concave lenses. Retinoscopy measures the refractive errors only and cannot determine the visual acuity.

377   a) False   b) False   c) True   d) False   e) False

Isotretinoin leads to CNS defects if given in the first trimester. Phenytoin leads to cleft lip, finger and toe abnormalities if given in the first trimester. Warfarin leads to neonatal haemorrhage if given in the third trimester. Given in the first trimester, it leads to nasal bone hypoplasia and bone defects in limbs. Sodium valproate, given in the first trimester, leads to neural tube defects.

378   a) False   b) False   c) False   d) True   e) True

The bullous form of impetigo is usually caused by Staphylococci and the non-bullous form by Streptococci. Atopic eczema is a predisposing factor. The crusts can be removed gently with cotton wool soaked in saline. Because of beta-lactamase–producing strains, bullous impetigo is usually treated by local fusidin or systemic amoxycillin-clavulanate (Augmentin).

379   a) True   b) True   c) True   d) True   e) True

380   a) True   b) False   c) True   d) True   e) False

381   a) False   b) True   c) False   d) True   e) False

Vaccines should be stored in refrigerators, but not in the door compartments. Vaccines despatched by post should not be accepted if 48 hours have elapsed since posting. Domestic refrigerators are generally inadequate for vaccine storage.

382 a) True   b) False   c) True   d) False   e) True

There is no justification to repeat the length measurement for all infants again and again. The weight should be repeatedly measured if clinically indicated or if the parents would like to do so.

383 a) True   b) True   c) True   d) False   e) True

Rotavirus is a common cause of gastroenteritis.

384 a) True   b) False   c) False   d) True   e) False

About 95% of all values lie between −2 SD and +2 SD. Thus, about 2.5% lie to the right of +2 SD and about 2.5% lie to the left of −2 SD. About 70% of all values lie between −1 SD and +1 SD. Prepubertal height follows such a distribution closely. This is probably due to the importance of genetic determinants. The prepubertal weight, on the other hand, does not follow a normal distribution closely, due to the importance of environmental factors.

385 a) False   b) True   c) True   d) True   e) True

Doubling, two children on one bicycle, is dangerous.

386 a) False   b) True   c) False   d) False   e) True

Most children can scribble spontaneously and build a tower of 3 cubes at 18 months. Most can turn pages singly at 2 years.

387 a) True   b) True   c) True   d) False   e) True

A high urine/plasma urea ratio is suggestive of pre-renal failure.

388 a)   True   b) True   c) True   d) False   e) True

Many methods have been designed for asthma screening, e.g. identifying 'keywords' in the GP notes, questionnaires, peakflowmetry, skin testing, IgE levels and exercise provocation. However, none fulfils Wilson and Jungner's criteria as justifiable and cost-effective screening tests for routine use on all children. There is no justification to repeat the testicular examination routinely at 18 to 24 months.

389 a) True   b) False   c) False   d) False   e) True

390 a) True   b) True   c) True   d) True   e) False

391   a) True   b) True   c) False   d) False   e) True

A 3-year-old child is too young to use powder inhalers. He should be at least 5 before powder inhalers can be used. The combination of a metered dose inhaler with a valved spacer is suitable from the age of 2 to 99! Although a 10-year-old child can use a metered dose inhaler by itself after adequate training, it is not advisable because there is much oropharyngeal deposition. If he is using regular prophylactic steroids, it is best to use a dry powder device (discs, turbuhaler or accuhaler) or an MDI with a valved spacer.

392   a) False   b) False   c) True   d) False   e) True

A herald patch, a 'T-shirt and shorts' distribution, peripheral scaling lesions and an 'inverted Christmas-tree' pattern are characteristic features of pityriasis rosea. About 50% of the presented cases have mild to moderate itch. However, as many cases are undiagnosed, pruritus is not a characteristic feature.

Pityriasis versicolor presents with round or oval lesions with margins not sharply defined. It may be hyper- or hypo-pigmented (*versi*color) and some pigment is usually still present. The above features distinguish it from vitiligo. It may sometimes be itchy, but this is not a characteristic feature.

Papular urticaria is not a type of 'urticaria'. It presents with localized clusters of papules due to insect or flea bites on the extremities of children. The lesions are intensely itchy.

Pityriasis alba is depigmentation and scaling on the face or limbs of children after atopic eczema or other causes of dermatitis. Itch is possible but uncommon.

Nodular prurigo is very itchy and can begin an itch-scratch cycle with surrounding patches of lichen simplex.

393   a) False   b) True   c) True   d) True   e) True

394   a) False   b) True   c) False   d) True   e) False

Ocular problems cause a pendular nystagmus. Vestibular problems cause a postural nystagmus. Cerebellar and brain stem lesions cause a phasic nystagmus.

395   a) False   b) False   c) True   d) True   e) False

Distant vision is tested at 6 m. Linear charts give a lower score due to the crowding phenomenon and are more sensitive for children with amblyopia. Diagrams can replace letters for small children as long as they can cooperate and the kits are standard. Near vision is tested at 25 cm.

396 a) True   b) False   c) False   d) False   e) False

For viral warts, spontaneous remission in 2 years is likely. Lesions on the faces of children should not be treated with electrocautery as it will result in ugly scars. Facial lesions should either be left untouched or treated with liquid nitrogen. Keratolytic agents will decrease the bulk of the lesion. If the wart totally disappears after the application and does not recur, spontaneous remission is likely to have occurred. Most children, upon careful explanation, tolerate cryosurgery surprisingly well.

397 a) True   b) False   c) False   d) False   e) False

398 a) True   b) True   c) True   d) False   e) True

Duodenal ulcer may lead to projectile vomiting if it leads to obstruction. The vomiting in gastroenteritis is not characteristically projectile.

399 a) False   b) True   c) True   d) False   e) True

400 a) True   b) False   c) False   d) False   e) True

Most children with neuroblastomata are below 2 years of age. If the lesion does not cross the midline of the abdomen, it can be both neuroblastoma or nephroblastoma. If it crosses the midline, it is more likely to be a neuroblastoma. Pallor, weight loss and calcifications seen in the ultrasound are features of neuroblastomata.

401 a) True   b) True   c) False   d) False   e) False

The decision to put the child on the Child Protection Register is made by the social service chair. According to the Children Act 1989, parents and young people can attend the case conference.

402 a) False   b) True   c) False   d) True   e) False

403 a) False   b) True   c) True   d) True   e) True

90% of all children with migraine have a family history. In girls, migraine attacks may be exacerbated in the premenstrual period, as part of the premenstrual syndrome.

404 a) True   b) True   c) True   d) True   e) True

405 a) True   b) True   c) True   d) True   e) False

Macroglossia in Beckwith's syndrome and a small mouth in Down's syndrome may lead to dysarthria. Only very rarely is tongue tie implicated as a cause of dysarthria.

406 a) True   b) False   c) True   d) False   e) True

124

407   a) True   b) False   c) True   d) True   e) True

408   a) True   b) False   c) True   d) True   e) True

409   a) False   b) False   c) True   d) False   e) False

The mid-parental height of a boy =

$$\frac{\text{Height of father} + \text{height of mother} + 12\ \text{cm}}{2}$$

The mid-parental height of a girl =

$$\frac{\text{Height of father} + \text{height of mother} - 12\ \text{cm}}{2}$$

The expected range of the final adult height =
mid-parental height ± 8 cm

410   a) True   b) False   c) False   d) True   e) True

Exacerbation by psychological stress suggests tension headache, periodic syndrome or migraine. Precipitation by cheese, chocolate, cherries or red wine suggests migraine. Aggravation by coughing suggests intracranial lesion.

411   a) True   b) False   c) True   d) True   e) True

The mother with HBsAg +ve, HBeAg –ve and HBeAb +ve has low infectivity. Hepatitis B vaccine but not immunoglobulin should be given to the baby. The mother with HBsAg –ve, HBsAb +ve and total anti-HBc –ve has already been successfully vaccinated against hepatitis B. The mother with HBsAg +ve, total HBcAb +ve and HBeAgAb unknown might have high infectivity. For safety, both vaccination and immunoglobulin should be given to the baby. The mother with HBsAg +ve, HBeAg +ve and HBeAb –ve has high infectivity. Both vaccination and immunoglobulin should be given to the baby. The mother with HBsAg –ve, total anti-HBc +ve and IgM anti-HBc +ve 5 weeks before delivery has had active infection with hepatitis B. Both vaccination and immunoglobulin should be given.

412   a) False   b) True   c) True   d) True   e) True

Note that galactossaemia can cause both conjugated and unconjugated hyperbilirubinaemia.

413   a) False   b) True   c) True   d) True   e) False

Febrile convulsions occur at 6 months to 5 years. By definition, convulsions caused by CNS infections are not febrile convulsions.

414   a) False   b) True   c) True   d) False   e) True

Adrenal insufficiency and hypothyroidism are causes of a positive sweat test, not Cushing's disease or thyrotoxicosis.

415   a) True   b) True   c) False   d) False   e) False

Urgent referral is indicated if the head circumference is crossing the centiles upwards with signs suggestive of hydrocephalus. If the head circumference is crossing the centiles upwards with no sign of hydrocephalus, repeating the measurements over many months will only cause parental anxiety. Two more measurements can be taken over a 4-week period. After this a decision must be made. Either the child is to be declared as normal, or he should be referred for imaging and other investigations.
  The same is true for head circumference crossing the centiles downwards. Prolonged repeat measurements are not to be recommended. If the child is considered normal, no adverse comment should be expressed to the parents. If he is considered abnormal, or if there is any doubt, referral for further investigations is needed.

416   a) True   b) False   c) True   d) True   e) False

Bleeding disorders are uncommon. Tumours as a cause of epistaxis in childhood are rare.

417   a) False   b) False   c) False   d) False   e) True

An undiagnosed viral infection is more likely than a bacterial infection. Connective tissue diseases account for about 15% of all cases. About 12–15% will finally remain undiagnosed. Evidence should be actively sought for in Munchausen syndrome. Kawasaki is a possible but relatively rare diagnosis.

418   a) False   b) True   c) False   d) False   e) False

The normal paediatric dosages are: phenytoin 5 mg/kg/24 h orally, carbamazepine 10–20 mg/kg/24 h orally, ampicillin 50–100 mg/kg/24 h orally and paracetamol 75 mg/kg/24 h orally.

419   a) False   b) True   c) False   d) True   e) False

Breast milk contains 60% whey and 40% casein. Cows' milk contains 80% casein and 20% whey. 'Humanized' formulae contain 60% whey and 40% casein. The milk requirement for an average infant is 150 ml/kg, or 100–110 kcal/kg/day, as the energy value of milk is about 20 kcal/30 ml. In general, both breast-fed and bottle-fed babies should be fed on demand. However, most mothers find it more convenient to have a fixed schedule. One must be flexible and most families will find a compromise between the two.

420   a) False   b) False   c) True   d) True   e) False

Chin reaching only to the tip of the shoulder, full wrist flexion and incomplete knee flexion with hips fully flexed are characteristic findings in a term baby.

421 **For intradermal administration of vaccines:**

a) A 23 g needle is used
b) The needle should be inserted to a depth of about 5 mm
c) A raised bleb signifies that the needle should be removed and reinserted
d) Pain should be minimal
e) A bleb of 7 mm diameter signifies that about 0.1 ml is injected

422 **Problems of babies born to mothers with poorly controlled diabetes mellitus include:**

a) Convulsions
b) Hypercalcaemia
c) Anal atresia
d) Hypoglycaemia
e) Hyperbilirubinaemia

423 **The following behaviours signify serious disturbance of the child and psychiatric referral should be considered:**

a) Masturbation
b) Setting fire
c) School phobia
d) Parasuicide
e) Running off from home

424 **Causes of urinary frequency include:**

a) Urinary tract infection
b) Neurogenic bladder
c) Anxiety
d) Hypocalcaemia
e) Compulsive water drinking

425 **A 9-year-old girl has ptosis with muscle weakness. The weakness becomes progressively worse as the day goes by:**

a) The Tensilon test should be performed
b) Acetylcholine receptor antibodies should be measured
c) Hypothyroidism is often associated
d) Thymectomy is usually indicated soon after the diagnosis
e) Complications include myasthenic crisis, cholinergic crisis and mixed crisis

426 **In truncus arteriosus:**

a) A common artery arises from both ventricles
b) A low ventricular defect exists
c) The pulmonary arteries come from the left ventricle
d) Pulses are usually weak
e) Pulmonary oligaemia is characteristic

427 **Equipment needed in a child health clinic includes:**

a) 100s and 1000s
b) Ishihara plate test for colour blindness
c) Percentile charts
d) STYCAR charts and test cards
e) Wall measuring chart

428 **The following statements are true:**

a) A child may be born with a tooth
b) The first tooth may appear when the child is 14 months old
c) The time of teething is related to the development of the child
d) Deciduous teeth are shed earlier in girls than in boys
e) The first tooth to appear is usually the upper central incisor

429 **A 6-week-old baby can:**

a) Follow a dangling toy from one side to the other
b) Pull at his clothes
c) Watch the mother when she talks to him
d) Lift chin off couch when lying prone
e) Smile momentarily when the mother talks to him

430 **Carvenous haemangiomata:**

a) Are usually pre-malignant
b) Commonly lead to thrombocytopenia
c) Are associated with haemangiomata of internal organs
d) Lead to low-output cardiac failure
e) Lead to undergrowth of a limb

431 **A 30-month-old child has short stature. The following are absolute indications for referral:**

a) History of congestive heart failure
b) Non-organic failure to thrive suspected
c) Height below –2 SD
d) Wasting
e) Chronic diarrhoea

432 **A 9-year-old girl has had recurrent abdominal pain for 6 months and has lost 5 kg in that period. Initial investigations reveal a high ESR. The following diagnoses are likely:**

a) Duodenal ulcer
b) Crohn disease
c) Chronic appendicitis
d) Ulcerative colitis
e) Meckel's diverticulum

433 **The Galant reflex:**

a) Is demonstrated by holding the baby vertically
b) Is positive if stepping movements of the legs are regular
c) Appears at about 5 months
d) When present in the first month of life, suggests dystonia
e) Is usually symmetrical

434 **For the day care facilities:**

a) Overcrowding and lack of toys and stimulation are important problems in play-groups
b) Day nurseries are staffed by nursery nurses who have undergone a 2-year training programme
c) Family centres teach parenting skills and increase the self-esteem of parents
d) Mother and toddler groups cater for young children and the mothers and they often move on to a playgroup
e) The integration of education and social service provision is a current trend

435 **A 10-month-old baby can:**

a) Stand alone momentarily
b) Clap hands
c) Creep upstairs
d) Build a tower of 2 cubes
e) Wave bye-bye

436 **Duties of the school nurse include:**

a) Giving DTP and polio boosters at 15 years
b) Testing hearing at school entry
c) Referring children with problems to the general practitioner
d) Testing colour vision
e) Performing the Heaf test and giving BCG immunization at 13 years

437 **Characteristic features of sickle cell trait include:**

a) Splenomegaly
b) Jaundice
c) Anaemia
d) Positive sickle cell test
e) Sickle cells and target cells in the blood film

438 **A child with no history of febrile convulsion just had a fit on the first day of a febrile illness. Lumbar puncture is indicated if he is:**

a) 15 months old with neck stiffness
b) 15 months old with no neck stiffness
c) 21 months old with neck stiffness
d) 3 years old with convulsions lasting more than 20 minutes
e) 6 years old with no neck stiffness

439 **Common causes of acute diarrhoea include:**

a) Haemolytic uraemic syndrome
b) Kawasaki disease
c) Otitis media
d) Pneumonia
e) Food poisoning

440 **In the screening for congenital dislocation of the hips:**

a) The pathway of referral should be decided by the individual doctors doing the screening
b) The neonate should be examined within the first 48 hours
c) The examination should be repeated at 6 to 8 months
d) The Ortolani-Barlow manoeuvre should be repeated at 6 to 9 months
e) Gait abnormalities should be noted at the 18 to 24 month review

441 **The following statements are true:**

a) The auditory response cradle detects changes in the infant's head turns and body movements
b) The brain-stem-evoked response audiometry (BSERA) analyses the EEG signals in response to a series of clicks
c) BSERA results are simple and easy to interpret
d) The evoked otoacoustic emissions test (EOAE) detects acoustic responses produced by the cochlear hair cells
e) EOAE is generally easier and quicker than BSERA

442 **Glandular fever:**

a) Is usually caused by the Epstein-Barr virus (EBV)
b) Is not caused by cytomegalovirus (CMV)
c) When caused by EBV, has demonstrable heterophile antibodies in 90% of cases
d) Causes a rash in less than half of the patients given ampicillin
e) May have encephalitis as the sole presenting feature

443 **In cystic fibrosis:**

a) Male sexual function is generally impaired
b) Females have increased risk of spontaneous abortion
c) The chance of a sibling being affected is 1 in 4 for a normal male marrying a female with the disease
d) Carrier detection and antenatal diagnosis are available
e) The prevalence of diabetes mellitus is increasing

444 **Symptoms of anaphylaxis after administration of a vaccine include:**

a) Palpitations
b) Angiooedema
c) Stridor
d) Shortness of breath
e) Peripheral oedema

445 **For the screening of congenital heart diseases:**

a) The heart should be examined at birth and at the review at 6 to 8 weeks
b) Persistent bradycardia is of particular significance
c) The examination should be repeated at 6 to 9 months
d) The examination should be repeated at 18 to 24 months
e) An ECG and an echocardiogram should be done for every neonate with Down's syndrome routinely during the first few weeks of life

446 **A baby born at 34th weeks of gestation has tachypnoea with grunting 2 hours after birth. Chest X-ray shows bilateral opaque lung fields with an air bronchogram. The most likely diagnosis is:**

a) Congenital pneumonia
b) Idiopathic respiratory distress syndrome
c) Bronchopulmonary dysplasia
d) Meconium aspiration
e) Transient tachypnoea of the newborn

447 **The criteria for a diagnosis of Kawasaki disease include:**

a) Erythematous rash which may also be macular or multiform
b) Aneurysms of the coronary vessels
c) Fever for 3 or more days
d) Suppurative cervical lymphadenopathy
e) Oedema of the hands and feet with peeling of the skin of the fingertips

448 **The following associations in poisoning are true:**

a) Antihistamines and haematemesis
b) Amphetamine and convulsion
c) Opiates and large pupils
d) Tricyclic antidepressants and small pupils
e) Phenothiazines and arrhythmias

449 **A child has recurrent episodes of gastroenteritis and bronchopneumonia. He has low lymphocyte counts and very low immunoglobulin levels. The most likely diagnosis is:**

a) Hypogammaglobulinaemia
b) Severe combined immunodeficiency
c) AIDS
d) Chronic mucocutaneous candidiasis
e) Chronic granulomatous disease

450 **Adverse effects of phenytoin include:**

a) SLE-like rash
b) Teratogenicity
c) Lymphadenopathy
d) Gum hypertrophy
e) Ataxia

131

451 In anaemia in prematurity:

a) The early (4–6 weeks) anaemia is nutritional
b) The late (8–12 weeks) anaemia is haemolytic
c) Nutritional anaemia is usually hypochromic
d) Haemolytic anaemia may be due to folic acid deficiency
e) Haemolytic anaemia may be due to vitamin E deficiency

452 For an infant with a strong family history of atopy:

a) Breastfeeding should be insisted upon
b) Introduction of other foods should best be delayed
c) Soya-based infant formulae are non-allergenic
d) Follow-on formulae may be less allergenic than fresh cows' milk
e) A restriction diet should be under the supervision of both a paediatrician and a dietician

453 Causes of recurrent abdominal pain are:

a) Constipation
b) Urinary tract infection
c) Abdominal migraine
d) Epilepsy
e) Mesenteric adenitis

454 The Personal Child Health Records:

a) Are more widely used in developed countries
b) Will sooner or later be lost by most parents
c) Pose serious threats on confidentiality
d) Can replace records kept by general practitioners
e) Contain useful information on health education

455 Secondary causes of obesity include:

a) Cushing's syndrome
b) Hypothyroidism
c) Down's syndrome
d) Hyperparathyroidism
e) Prader–Willi syndrome

456 For necrotizing enterocolitis:

a) Term babies are particularly at risk
b) Perinatal asphyxia is a risk factor
c) Expressed breast milk from a milk bank confers no protection
d) Failure of temperature control is a late sign
e) High platelet count is frequently seen

457 In birth trauma:

a) Erb's palsy involves C6, C7 and C8
b) Klumpke's palsy involves C7, C8 and T1
c) Facial nerve palsy leads to a persistently closed eye
d) Sciatic nerve involvement is common
e) Cephalohaematoma is characteristically present at birth

458 Thrombocytopenia purpura:

a) Is not caused by aspirin
b) Is often preceded by a viral disease
c) Will lead to a prolonged APTT
d) Will lead to a prolonged PT
e) May be controlled by splenectomy

459 The following are contraindications to the pertussis vaccine:

a) Cerebral palsy
b) Severe local reactions to a previous dose
c) History of febrile convulsion
d) Evolving neurological problem
e) Family history of epilepsy

460 Café-au-lait patches are associated with:

a) Shagreen patches
b) Axillary freckles
c) Adenoma sebaceum
d) Premature puberty
e) Strawberry naevi

461 The following commonly cause ventricular premature beats:

a) Myocarditis
b) Digoxin
c) Hypercalcaemia
d) Hypocalcaemia
e) Hypokalaemia

462 Equipment needed in a child health clinic includes:

a) Child health record cards
b) 1-inch (2.5 cm) cubes
c) MEG warbler
d) Toys for distraction test
e) Cup-and-spoon

463 **Causes of recurrent abdominal pain include:**

a) Diabetes mellitus
b) Lead poisoning
c) Hypoglycaemia
d) Recurrent pancreatitis
e) C1-esterase inhibitor deficiency

464 **In CSF microscopy:**

a) Gram-negative cocci suggest *Haemophilus influenzae*
b) Gram-negative intracellular diplococci suggest meningococci
c) Gram-positive bacilli suggest pneumococci
d) Gram-positive intracellular diplococci suggest meningococci
e) The diagnosis should always be confirmed by culture before treatment

465 **The following are contraindications of emesis in the management of poisoning:**

a) More than 4 hours after ingestion of paraquat
b) More than 4 hours after ingestion of aspirin
c) Ingestion of volatile liquids
d) Ingestion of corrosive liquids
e) A conscious child crying actively

466 **A neonate has just been confirmed to have Down's syndrome:**

a) The diagnosis should first be suggested to the parents by a nurse, then confirmed by a paediatrician
b) The parents should be informed several weeks later so that good parental bonds are formed
c) Both parents should be informed together
d) The prediction of future disabilities and complications should be extensively described to the parents
e) A second interview should be arranged about 24 hours later

467 **Causes of haematuria include:**

a) Myoglobinuria
b) Phenazopyridine
c) Beeturia
d) Dyes
e) Haemolytic anaemia

468 **Features in families with child abuse include:**

a) Single parents
b) Young parents
c) Extended family network
d) Living in deprived areas
e) Father with criminal record

469 The following favour a diagnosis of nephritis rather than nephrosis:

a) Unknown cause
b) Pre-school age
c) Sudden onset
d) Normal C3 complement
e) Hypercholesterolaemia

470 Common causes of constipation include:

a) Hirschprung's disease
b) Hypocalcaemia
c) Hypercalcaemia
d) Thyrotoxicosis
e) Hypothyroidism

471 Causes of growth-hormone-related short stature include:

a) CNS infection
b) Hypochondroplasia
c) Noonan's syndrome
d) Craniopharyngioma
e) Malabsorption

472 In dehydration:

a) A child who is 5% dehydrated has a sunken anterior fontanelle
b) A child who is 5% dehydrated usually has reduced skin turgor
c) A child who is 10% dehydrated usually has sunken eyes
d) A child who is 10% dehydrated usually has a dry tongue
e) For rapid correction of 10% dehydration, colloid solutions should be used

473 The Emergency Protection Order:

a) Confers parental responsibility
b) Prevents the child from removal from a hospital or foster home or removes the child from a dangerous situation
c) Lasts for 1 month
d) Does not allow the parents to make an appeal
e) Can direct a psychiatric examination to take place

474 The following congenital conditions require immediate (within the first week) treatment after birth:

a) Tracheo-oesophageal fistula
b) Cleft lip
c) Spina bifida
d) Exomphalos
e) Hydrocephalus

475   **For a child with food refusal:**

a) Snacks should be given to prevent the child from hunger
b) If the child eats, rewards should be given as a reinforcement
c) If the child does not eat anything, his plate should be taken away
d) Grandparents are usually helpful in the management
e) The anxiety of the mother should be appropriately managed

476   **Indications for circumcision include:**

a) Ballooning
b) Balanitis with pus formation
c) Balanitis xerotica obliterans
d) Long foreskin
e) The parents are distressed and request for the operation

477   **Conditions associated with polyhydramnios include:**

a) Oesophageal atresia
b) Down's syndrome
c) Renal agenesis
d) Cord around the neck
e) CNS malformation

478   **A 7-year-old girl with polyuria has urine osmolality of 870 mmol/l, 8 hours after water deprivation. Her usual plasma and urine osmolalities are low. The most likely diagnosis is:**

a) Compulsive water drinking
b) Diabetes mellitus
c) Central diabetes insipidus
d) Nephrogenic diabetes insipidus
e) Chronic renal failure

479   **Hazards of exchange transfusion include:**

a) Hypercalcaemia
b) Haemorrhage
c) Hypothermia
d) Infection
e) Hyperglycaemia

480   **In pauci-articular JCA:**

a) ESR is elevated
b) C-reactive protein is elevated
c) Albumin: globulin ratio is commonly reversed
d) Selective IgA deficiency is associated
e) Most will resolve by 16 years of age

| **421** | **a) False** | **b) False** | **c) False** | **d) False** | **e) True** |

A 25 g or 26 g needle is to be used for the intradermal administration of vaccines such as BCG. The needle should be injected almost horizontally, to a depth of about 2 mm. A raised bleb is a sign that the injection has been successful. The procedure is quite painful.

| **422** | **a) True** | **b) False** | **c) True** | **d) True** | **e) True** |

| **423** | **a) False** | **b) True** | **c) False** | **d) True** | **e) True** |

| **424** | **a) True** | **b) True** | **c) True** | **d) False** | **e) True** |

In general, causes of urinary obstruction can cause frequency. Hypercalcaemia is a cause of urinary frequency due to polyuria. Hypocalcaemia is not a cause.

| **425** | **a) True** | **b) True** | **c) False** | **d) False** | **e) True** |

IV endrophonium improves the weakness in myasthenia gravis rapidly and this is the Tensilon test. Hyperthyroidism may be associated. Thymectomy is rarely indicated in children.

| **426** | **a) True** | **b) False** | **c) False** | **d) False** | **e) False** |

The VSD in truncus arteriosus is high. The pulmonary arteries arise from the truncus itself, not from the left ventricle. The pulse is collapsing and pulmonary plethora is characteristic.

| **427** | **a) True** | **b) False** | **c) True** | **d) True** | **e) True** |

Testing for defects in colour vision is not routinely undertaken in a child health clinic. The school health service is generally responsible for testing, if facilities for career advice or referral is available.

| **428** | **a) True** | **b) True** | **c) False** | **d) False** | **e) False** |

Deciduous teeth are shed earlier in boys than in girls. The first tooth to appear is usually the lower central incisor.

| **429** | **a) False** | **b) False** | **c) True** | **d) True** | **e) True** |

Most babies can follow a dangling object from one side to the other and pull at his clothes at 3 months.

| **430** | **a) False** | **b) False** | **c) True** | **d) False** | **e) False** |

Carvenous haemangiomata are benign. Thrombocytopenia is possible but uncommon. Large haemangiomata can lead to high-output cardiac failure. It can also lead to the overgrowth of a limb.

431   **a) True**   **b) True**   **c) False**   **d) True**   **e) True**

A height below –3 SD is an indication for referral by itself.

432   **a) False**   **b) True**   **c) False**   **d) True**   **e) False**

433   **a) False**   **b) False**   **c) False**   **d) False**   **e) True**

The Galant reflex is demonstrated by holding the baby in ventral suspension. Stroking the back with fingernails will lead to flexion of the spine to the stimulated side. The reflex is a primary reflex and is present at birth.

434   **a) False**   **b) True**   **c) True**   **d) True**   **e) True**

Overcrowding and lack of toys and stimulation are typical problems of childminders.

435   **a) False**   **b) True**   **c) False**   **d) False**   **e) True**

Most babies cannot stand alone momentarily at 10 months (although some can). Most can creep upstairs at 15 months and build a tower of 2 cubes at 1 year. Most can wave bye-bye at 10 months, although some babies manage to do this only at 1 year.

436   **a) False**   **b) True**   **c) True**   **d) True**   **e) True**

Td is now given, not DPT, at 15 years. The 'sweep test' is the hearing screening test done at school entry. It is usually performed by the school nurse or an audiologist. The Heaf test is done by the school nurse or the school doctor.

437   **a) False**   **b) False**   **c) False**   **d) True**   **e) True**

438   **a) True**   **b) True**   **c) True**   **d) True**   **e) True**

The presence of meningeal signs such as neck rigidity is, of course, an indication for lumbar puncture. Lumbar puncture is also indicated for any child below 18 months of age having the first convulsion, even if no added feature is present. For the 3-year-old child with convulsions lasting more than 15 minutes, it is also best to proceed to lumbar puncture if this is the first fit in his life. Lumbar puncture is indicated for any child with the first fit older than 5 years.

439   **a) False**   **b) False**   **c) True**   **d) True**   **e) True**

Haemolytic uraemic syndrome and Kawasaki disease are associated with acute diarrhoea, which typically occurs during the prodromal phase of the two diseases. However, these two diseases are uncommon.

440   a) False   b) True   c) False   d) False   e) True

The pathway for referral for any screening programme should be clearly defined beforehand. The examination should be repeated at 6 to 8 weeks. The most effective procedure at 6 to 9 months is to examine for limited abduction and asymmetry of the skin creases.

441   a) True   b) True   c) False   d) True   e) True

442   a) True   b) False   c) False   d) False   e) True

CMV and EBV can cause an identical disease. Heterophile antibodies can be demonstrated in about 50–60% of cases of glandular fever caused by EBV. More than half will exhibit a rash if ampicillin is given.

443   a) False   b) True   c) False   d) True   e) True

Cystic fibrosis is autosomal recessive. Two carriers will give a risk of 1 in 4 for an affected sibling. The prevalence of diabetes mellitus in cystic fibrosis is increasing. This might reflect an increasing lifespan of the patients. More than 95% of males are azoospermic, but sexual function is generally unimpaired.

444   a) True   b) True   c) True   d) True   e) True

The palpitations are due to hypotension in the anaphylactic shock. Both upper and lower airway obstruction can be present.

445   a) True   b) False   c) False   d) False   e) True

Persistent tachycardia is of particular significance. The examination should be repeated at 6 to 9 months or later only if there are relevant complaints or the child is examined for other reasons.

446   a) False   b) True   c) False   d) False   e) False

447   a) True   b) False   c) False   d) False   e) True

Aneurysms of the coronary vessels are an occasional complication and is not a diagnostic criterion. Fever for 5 or more days and non-suppurative cervical lymphadenopathy are diagnostic criteria. Other criteria are: conjunctivitis, dry and cracked lips with strawberry tongue. More than five features are needed to make a diagnosis. Three features make a diagnosis of atypical disease.

448   a) False   b) True   c) False   d) False   e) True

Opiates are associated with pinpoint pupils. The pupils are large in tricyclic antidepressant poisoning due to the anticholinergic effect.

449   a) False   b) True   c) False   d) False   e) False

The lymphocyte count in hypogammaglobulinaemia is normal. In AIDS, the T-helper cells are affected. In chronic mucocutaneous candidiasis, T-cells are affected and the immunoglobulin level is normal. Phagocytes are affected in chronic granulomatous disease and the immunoglobulin level is normal.

450   a) True   b) True   c) True   d) True   e) True

Phenytoin is a cause of drug-induced LE. It causes the phenytoin syndrome in infants.

451   a) False   b) False   c) True   d) True   e) True

The early (4–6 weeks) anaemia in premature infants is dilutional. The late (8–12 weeks) anaemia is usually nutritional.

452   a) False   b) True   c) False   d) True   e) True

One cannot insist but can only encourage the mother to breastfeed. Soya-based formulae may also be allergenic.

453   a) True   b) True   c) True   d) True   e) True

454   a) False   b) False   c) False   d) False   e) True

The Personal Child Health Record (PCHR) is more widely used in developing countries. Most parents will not lose the PCHR. There is usually no conflict with confidentiality as the parents decide who has access to the PCHR. General practitioners must keep their own records as one of their terms of service.

455   a) True   b) True   c) True   d) False   e) True

456   a) False   b) True   c) False   d) False   e) False

Preterm babies are particularly at risk of necrotizing enterocolitis. The failure of temperature control is an early sign. Thrombocytopenia may be present.

457   a) False   b) True   c) False   d) False   e) False

Erb's palsy involves C5 and C6. Facial nerve palsy leads to a persistently open eye. Sciatic nerve involvement is rare. If affected, S1–S4 will be involved with foot drop. Cephalohaematoma is usually obvious at 2 to 5 days old.

458   a) False   b) True   c) False   d) False   e) True

Aspirin can lead to both thrombocytopenia and platelet function abnormalities. APTT is not prolonged in thrombocytopenia purpura as the intrinsic pathway is not affected. The PT is also normal as the extrinsic pathway is not affected.

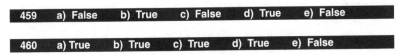

| **459** | a) False | b) True | c) False | d) True | e) False |

| **460** | a) True | b) True | c) True | d) True | e) False |

Shagreen patches and adenoma sebaceum are seen in tuberous sclerosis. Axillary freckles are seen in neurofibromatosis-1. Premature puberty is a feature in McCune–Albright syndrome. All these diseases are associated with café-au-lait patches.

| **461** | a) True | b) True | c) True | d) False | e) False |

Hypercalcaemia and hyperkalaemia are causes of ventricular premature beats.

| **462** | a) True | b) True | c) True | d) True | e) False |

The cup-and-spoon is no longer recommended as a sound source for the distraction test.

| **463** | a) True | b) True | c) True | d) True | e) True |

| **464** | a) False | b) True | c) False | d) False | e) False |

Haemophilus influenzae are gram negative coccobacilli. Pneumococci are gram positive diplococci. Treatment should be started on a best-guess approach as soon as possible and modified when the culture results are available.

| **465** | a) True | b) False | c) True | d) True | e) False |

More than 12 hours after ingestion of aspirin is a contraindication to emesis. Unconsciousness is also a contraindication.

| **466** | a) False | b) False | c) True | d) False | e) True |

A senior member of the team, e.g. the consultant paediatrician, should inform the parents, preferably with the health visitor. They should be informed as soon as possible. It might be too cruel to describe complications such as dementia, atlanto-axial subluxation or leukaemia to the parents at this point. Major implications, e.g. that the child might not be able to attain higher education, should be described in a conservative but optimistic manner. A second interview is necessary to consolidate the information and to answer questions.

| **467** | a) False | b) False | c) False | d) False | e) False |

| **468** | a) True | b) True | c) False | d) True | e) True |

The lack of extended family support is a risk factor.

469   **a) False**   **b) False**   **c) True**   **d) False**   **e) False**

Both nephritis and nephrosis can have unknown cause. Nephrosis occurs mainly in pre-school children. Normal C3 complement and hypercholesterolaemia are also characteristic features of nephrosis.

470   **a) False**   **b) False**   **c) False**   **d) False**   **e) False**

Hirschprung's disease can cause both constipation and diarrhoea. However, it is uncommon. Hypocalcaemia does not cause constipation. Hypercalcaemia does. However, it is also uncommon. Thyrotoxicosis causes diarrhoea. Hypothyroidism causes constipation. However, with the current screening programme this ought to be an uncommon cause.

471   **a) True**   **b) False**   **c) False**   **d) True**   **e) False**

472   **a) True**   **b) False**   **c) False**   **d) True**   **e) True**

A sunken anterior fontanelle is one of the early signs of dehydration. Reduced skin turgor signifies 10–15% dehydration. Sunken eyes signify at least 15% dehydration and is a late sign.

473   **a) True**   **b) True**   **c) False**   **d) False**   **e) True**

The Emergency Protection Order confers parental responsibility during the period covered by the order. Its main use is to detain the child temporarily for investigations to take place. It is effective for 8 days initially, and can then be renewed for a further 7 days. The child or the parents can appeal after 72 hours.

474   **a) True**   **b) False**   **c) True**   **d) True**   **e) False**

475   **a) False**   **b) False**   **c) True**   **d) False**   **e) True**

Giving snacks will only further worsen the appetite. Bribes should not be given. Grandparents usually make the matter worse by forcefeeding or giving snacks. They create unnecessary anxiety for the parents. Food refusal is an example in which the whole family should be treated together, not only the child.

476   **a) False**   **b) True**   **c) True**   **d) False**   **e) False**

477   **a) True**   **b) True**   **c) False**   **d) True**   **e) True**

Renal agenesis leads to oligohydramnios.

478	a) True	b) False	c) False	d) False	e) False

479	a) False	b) True	c) True	d) True	e) False

Hypocalcaemia is a hazard due to the citrate in preserved blood binding the calcium. Haemorrhage is often due to tubing disconnection. Hypoglycaemia is a recognised risk.

480	a) True	b) False	c) True	d) True	e) True

C-reactive protein is usually normal in pauciarticular JCA. Elevation suggests a bacterial infection.

SUBJECT INDEX

The numbers given are question numbers

CARDIOLOGY

6 25 58 75 106 130 155 162 175 177 180 182 189 196
200 203 205 210 256 267 299 355 358 389 426 445 461

COMMUNITY PAEDIATRICS

3 5 8 15 17 33 43 53 63 66 81 90 99 107 109 111 126
154 163 164 165 168 169 171 174 199 208 216 218 227
243 253 258 259 263 276 292 301 304 314 315 317 320
321 323 327 330 335 339 342 343 365 372 379 382 385
388 401 404 427 434 436 454 462 468 473

DERMATOLOGY

13 27 30 79 84 140 190 214 238 255 331 350 357 378
392 396 430 460

ENDOCRINOLOGY AND METABOLIC DISORDERS

11 21 22 41 45 77 134 139 173 197 213 271 287 329 333
412 414 422 443 455 470 471 478

EPIDEMIOLOGY AND CLINICAL AUDIT

258 300 309 362 374 384

GASTROENTEROLOGY AND NUTRITION

20 39 50 64 69 72 101 114 115 132 151 152 183 187 193
195 215 247 280 285 294 305 308 316 322 330 340 345
373 398 402 419 428 432 439 452 453 456 463 470 472

GENETICS

26 65 73 82 93 94 103 131 176 197 211 281 443 466

GENITO-URINARY MEDICINE

1 116 123 217 248 291 298 319 361 367 408 476

GROWTH AND DEVELOPMENT

4 16 18 54 64 66 77 100 105 118 146 159 197 201 221

PSYCHIATRY AND BEHAVIOUR

31 80 95 113 143 150 153 164 233 254 295 296 302 324
325 423 475 478

RESPIRATORY DISEASES

10 28 42 68 133 135 161 170 177 181 200 206 212 229
236 237 242 288 290 332 337 345 351 383 391 414 446

RHEUMATOLOGY AND ORTHOPAEDICS

38 121 142 167 178 251 272 289 349 353 370 440 480

THERAPEUTICS

61 89 101 113 114 128 137 172 188 195 294 356 377 402
418 450

INDEX

The numbers given are question numbers.
The term shown may not always be used in
the question but may appear in the
explanatory notes.

Index

Index

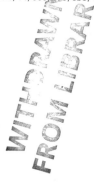

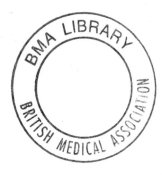